The Prostate Health Diet

What to Eat to Prevent and Heal Prostate Problems

Including Prostate Cancer, BPH Enlarged Prostatitis

Ronald M. Bazar

BCom, McGill University

MBA, Harvard University

The Prostate Health Diet

What to Eat to Prevent and Heal Prostate Problems Including Prostate Cancer, BPH Enlarged Prostate and Prostatitis

Author:
Ronald M. Bazar
BCom, McGill University
MBA, Harvard University

Published by:
Ronald M. Bazar, PO Box 73, Mansons Landing, BC V0P 1K0 Canada

Email: healthyprostate@ymail.com

First Edition: May 2013
Copyright © 2013 by Ronald M. Bazar
ISBN: 978-1490484099
All Rights Reserved

www.ProstateHealthDiet.org

Acknowledgements

I thank Coreen Boucher at Lucent Edits, who again has come to my rescue to make this book as smooth flowing and readable as could be done!

The Prostate Health Diet

Dear Reader,

I have written this book to help guide you through the maze of information that you will find about diets that focus on prostate health. There is much to learn about what is good for your prostate and what harms it.

Too much information about diets invades our lives and much of it is contradictory! Well-meaning advisors often have a particular diet that worked for them, and they think that they have found the answer for everyone. Others center their diets on "scientific findings" that are often based on critical assumptions, which turn out to be incorrect.

So how are you to know what to do? And why is this diet book any different from those I critique?

I will teach you how to find what works for you, and it will be customized for your unique body. There is no one diet for everyone!

In my quest to heal my enlarged prostate condition without drugs or surgery, I tried all kinds of excellent advice—or so I thought—and it didn't work!

It wasn't until later on, after 8 years, that I finally discovered the lessons and secrets to success that I am going to share with you here.

I have already written a successful book on that experience and my quest called *Healthy Prostate: The Extensive Guide To Prevent and Heal Prostate Problems Including Prostate Cancer, BPH Enlarged Prostate and Prostatitis*.

However, this book is a simpler, shorter book that focuses on diet and distills the important information about diet so you can prevent prostate problems in the first place and can heal them if you have a condition.

Our diets, in the broad sense of the word, include all of our inputs and are the single most important issue to ensure our health and our prostate health in particular. Why? Because the prostate gland has many important functions.

Perhaps its most crucial one is to protect the sperm from toxins by removing them and storing them in the prostate itself. Those toxins then affect your prostate health and can lead to prostate disease.

Because of the avalanche of toxins in our modern diets, prostate conditions have exploded in the West over the past decades to a level that will affect most men at some point in their lives.

You can ignore that sad state of affairs or be proactive in prevention. I wish I knew decades ago what you are about to read here!

To your good health!
Ron Bazar

Introduction

How wonderful it is to be young! Our bodies are strong. We can eat whatever we want and feel no side effects.

And then we get older, turning the 40s hump and then the 50s and things start to catch up with us. Now we start to feel the effects of so many tiny decisions of yesteryear. Chronic health conditions arise and affect us by making our lives much more difficult.

In men, we start to feel the effects of changing testosterone levels: lower libido, poor staying power and get up and go difficulties. Our prostates, which are command central for our sexual health and potency, feel the ravages of time. Sexual difficulties arise. We find ourselves worrying about our prostates, wondering if prostate cancer—the primary cancer in men—will invade our lives.

We wake up at night ever more often to pee. Some men start to have other symptoms of an enlarged prostate like dribbling, hesitancy, frequency and difficulty voiding. Our lives are impacted as we always need to know where the washroom is if we are away from home.

Given the industrialization of our food supply and the poor eating habits of a lifetime, it is no wonder that prostate disease has skyrocketed in the U.S. and the Western modern world. Traditional cultures do not have the sky-high rates of prostate conditions that we do. So the master of time and the unaware choices we have made have finally caught up with us.

Your prostate health is in your hands, not your doctor's. Sadly, most men will follow the dictates of their MD or urologist when it comes to their prostate. They never fully understand how they got their prostate condition, nor how to reverse it naturally.

The Prostate Health Diet focuses on your health, your diet and the choices you make every day. My goal is to help you become very educated about the "food" you eat in the broadest definition of that term (i.e., all of your inputs) so you can make much better informed decisions. This way you can achieve a much healthier prostate and an overall higher quality of health.

The bad news is that there is no shortcut. You need to learn about the impact of your daily food choices and make better decisions for your health. It will challenge your lifestyle. It will ask you to make changes.

In this book, I include a scale of diets, from poorest to optimum. You may think that I go too far, but in reality, humans have gone too far astray in our food production and diet choices. Our modern lifestyles have compromised our health so much that what I propose may seem extreme for many of you.

I suggest we eat a much simpler and more nourishing diet that will make sense to you if you have an open mind. No fads, no diet dictates, no gimmicks—just common sense and the knowledge that it is based on proven concepts. It's not founded on garbage science under the influence of special interests and deep pockets, or on well- intentioned health practitioners who think they know what you should eat!

The good news? Eating this way is no sacrifice. Food will be extremely tasty and delicious, not boring, bland, or yucky as so many fad diets propose.

For most men, there is much to learn for we have put diet low on our priority list for decades. You are at a turning point and, if you are open to embrace what I share with you here, not only will your prostate respond happily, but your overall health will be recharged. You will lose weight, feel a whole lot better and improve your sex life.

I am no jock born with the gifts of a strong constitution and great physique. Yet I have managed at this 66th year of my life to be in great shape, run, swim and play sports often with men much younger than me. I credit most of this to the attention I pay to my diet and the exercise that I do each week.

What I offer in *The Prostate Health Diet* are the tools to transform your health so this next phase of your life can be the best possible time for you. Are you ready to learn and to make changes? Then this book is for you. Read on!

Official Disclaimer & Legal Notice

The statements in this book have not been evaluated by the Food and Drug Administration (FDA) or any other government agency of any country. Nothing in this book is intended to treat, cure or prevent any disease. The information presented is not intended to replace the advice of your doctor.

This book is for informational and educational purposes only and is not a substitute for medical advice, diagnosis or treatment provided by a qualified health care provider. It is offered as research and personal opinion to help you understand your current situation and to help you expand your knowledge as a more informed participant in your health choices. You and you alone are responsible for what you do.

Please see your physician before changing your diet, doing a cleanse or treatment, starting a new exercise program, or taking any dietary herbs or supplements of any kind, or following any of the advice or suggestions in this book. Seek the advice of a qualified natural health professional to supplement the advice of your doctor. Make your own health care decisions based upon your own research and in partnership with your physician.

The views and statements expressed in this book represent the opinion of the author and should not be considered scientific or medical conclusions. The author does not assume any liability for the information contained herein. Specific medical advice should be obtained from a licensed health care practitioner.

As the reader, you agree that no responsibility or liability will be incurred to the author with respect to any loss, damage or injury caused or alleged to be caused directly or indirectly by the information contained herein. **If you do not agree to this statement, then please do not read this book!** If you have a severe medical condition, please see a licensed healthcare practitioner.

Ron

Contents

Chapter 1: The Prostate and How it Works

Do you know the 10 amazing functions of the prostate gland? No wonder it is so vital to men's health and the propagation of the species

The Prostate's Purpose

Gland

The primary job of the prostate is to produce and secrete some of the alkaline seminal fluids during ejaculation (about 30 to 35% of the semen ejaculate). Being alkaline, the prostate fluid, which is milky whitish in color, helps the sperm survive in the acidic vaginal environment. The prostate is considered to be a gland since glands secrete something.

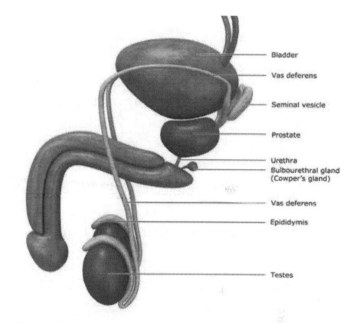

Mix Master

The prostate mixes its fluids with those from the seminal vesicles to transport the sperm made in the testicles. Together these fluids surge through the prostate into the urethra during ejaculation. The urethra doubles as the semen tube during ejaculation and as the urine tube from the bladder, both fluids exiting the tip of the penis (at different times!). The section of the urethra that runs through the prostate gland is called the prostatic urethra and is about 3cm (1½") long.

Prostate-specific antigen (PSA) is a fluid produced in the prostate, playing a key role in enabling the sperm to swim into the uterus by keeping the semen in liquid form. It counteracts the clotting enzyme in the seminal vesicle fluid, which essentially glues the semen to the woman's cervix, next to the uterus entrance inside the vagina. PSA dissolves this glue with its own enzyme so that the sperm can dash into the uterus and impregnate an egg if it is there.

It is this same PSA that is tested during the PSA blood test, a very controversial test because of the many factors that can cause the results to vary widely.

Muscle

The prostate is also a muscle that pumps the semen out through the penis with enough force to enter into the vagina to help the sperm succeed in reaching the cervix and ensuring procreation of the species.

AH!

An added bonus for males, the pumping action of the prostate sure feels good, making sex desirable and thus helping procreation.

G-spot

The prostate is the male G-spot. Prostate stimulation can produce an exceptionally strong sexual response and intense orgasm in men that are receptive to this sexual technique. The ability to control ejaculation at the prostate can also lead to prolonged orgasms and "injaculations" where no semen is expelled. This is done in advanced Taoist and Tantric sexual practices to contain the sexual energy internally.

Filter

The prostate also filters and removes toxins for protection of the sperm, which enhances the chance of impregnation and ensures that men seed with the optimum quality of sperm. This is perhaps the prostate's most important function and, at the same time, can be one of the main reasons there is a growing epidemic of prostate disease and cancer as men deal with more and more toxins in food and the environment.

Erections

The prostate erection nerves are responsible for erections. These nerves trigger the penis to swell and harden with extra blood flow into it, producing an erection.

If these nerves, which attach to the sides of the prostate, get damaged then erectile difficulties are guaranteed. That is why many medical prostate procedures (surgery or radiation) have an unwanted side effect of erectile difficulties or impotence.

Secretions

Prostatic secretions also play a valuable role by protecting the urethra from urinary tract infections, which seem to be much rarer in men than women.

Valves

The prostate surrounds the upper part of the urethra tube just below the bladder (the prostatic urethra) and controls the flow of urine. It prevents urine from leaving the bladder, except when released by urination. It also prevents urine from damaging ejaculate during orgasm.

It does this with two small prostatic muscles called sphincters. They act as gatekeepers with shut-off valves to control and regulate the dual-purpose urethra tube. These gatekeepers ensure the right fluids flow at the right time—urination or ejaculation. Not a bad design!

One sphincter is located where the bladder and the upper part of the prostate meet (the internal upper sphincter). When functioning properly, it prevents urination until it's time to go, and stops seminal fluid from shooting backwards into the bladder during ejaculation.

When this sphincter is damaged, semen is forced back into the bladder and eventually exits with normal urination. This is known as retrograde ejaculation and is another possible side effect of prostate surgery—no chance of seeding a woman then!

The second, external lower sphincter is at the base of the prostate and is subject to our control. It prevents dribbling after peeing and is how we voluntarily can delay urination when inconvenient to go. Incontinence occurs when control of either sphincter is damaged and urine leaks or flows uncontrollably, thus forcing many men with prostate problems to wear adult diapers.

It's easy enough to voluntarily control the lower sphincter and to stop urine or semen from exiting if you have enough Kegel muscle control, the ability to squeeze the flow shut. Either one of these sphincter muscles will block the urine until the urge to pee happens and the timing is right to release and let the urine flow.

An enlarged prostate or BPH can squeeze the prostatic urethra tube and the upper or lower sphincter, making urination difficult with a host of unpleasant, uncontrollable symptoms. BPH surgeries that remove part of the prostate can easily have side effects of incontinence or retrograde ejaculation.

Hormones

The prostate gland contains a crucial enzyme, 5-alpha-reductase. This enzyme converts the hormone testosterone in the body to DHT (dihydrotestosterone), which is at least ten times more powerful than simple testosterone. This potent hormone DHT has several purposes including male sexual drive and function. Over time, a build-up of toxins in the prostate may affect the production of this enzyme, which is then responsible for the declining sex drive in men as they age.

DHT and testosterone have mistakenly been targeted as guilty hormones in prostate problems rather than the excessive rise in modern male estrogen levels, leading often to medical interventions with serious side effects including lack of libido.

Estrogen levels rise because of the prevalence of estrogens in factory foods, commercial meats and dairy as well as estrogen-mimicking chemicals present in body-care and household products. It's even found in municipal water and some plastic food packaging.

With such a complex gland having so many functions, prostate disease can wreak havoc on a man's health. Men would be wise to do all they can to enhance the health of their prostate—an unhealthy prostate can have an enormous impact on sexual function and simple daily urination.

The prostate is a powerhouse: a remarkable gland with huge repercussions on a man's quality of life!

It's actually a brilliant design! This is contrary to the suggestion that many urologists have jokingly made about how the prostate should be somewhere else.

But just look again at its amazing functions. The prostate is awe-inspiring for its perfect design: on-off switches to control what comes out of the penis—urine or ejaculate at the right time. Otherwise we would need two separate organs. Imagine those complications—

one for sex and one for urination! I guess you could have two penises, but one would certainly get in the way at the wrong time!

No, we have a brilliant system. The problem arises when we have the wrong inputs and start to suffer from prostate conditions! All the prostate is doing is performing one of its key functions—eliminating toxins from the ejaculate to protect the sperm. Unfortunately that means health problems because we are inundated with toxins.

Remember how close the prostate is to the bladder and rectum. Your prostate can easily absorb toxins from these organs because of their proximity. That is why our diets, in the broad sense of the word, are so crucial to the health of the prostate.

> The urinary tract and rectum are organs through which most of the waste products and toxins in our body are eliminated. The higher the level of toxicity in a person's body, the higher the level of toxicity present in their urine and feces. The proximity of the prostate to these organs makes it very susceptible to an accumulation of toxicity — both as urine passes through the prostate, and as toxins leach out of urine stored in the bladder and feces stored in the rectum between bowel movements.
>
> Prostate Health: Herbs for Treating Inflammation by M. Vertolli, tiny.cc/j1xrzw

So what is the solution? Add more toxins in the form of meds with huge side effects and cancer risks? Or, in the case of cancer, radiate and chemicalize the poor prostate? Well, if you think that is the way to go, then you are fooling yourself, in my opinion.

First, you will get side effects of incontinence (dribbling and diapers) or impotence (troubles getting it up). Then because you are adding more trauma to your body, you will eventually get recurrence of conditions in the prostate. You can even get prostate cancer again if your prostate has been removed. Yes, the cancer will affect the area around where it once was.

The only solution that makes any sense to me is to stop the inputs and the real causes of your condition or best of all change now to prevent the awful prostate symptoms and conditions from arising in the first place.

Too much trouble to make changes? Then life will force changes on you at some point down the road. Health is the ultimate wealth. Without good health what are you left with? Good health is an investment with wonderful paybacks that profit you for the rest of your life—one lived in vitality rather than chronic health conditions.

So nourish your prostate. Eat wisely on all the dimensions of food we will discuss. Learn about whole real foods that will feed you with benefits.

To learn more about your prostate, the real causes of prostate disease and the way to reverse a prostate problem, please read more in my ebook for instant download *Healthy Prostate: The Extensive Guide to Prevent and Heal Prostate Problems* (www.healthyprostate.co/) or order as a print book from Amazon.

Conclusion

Once I understood that the prostate had so many vital functions, I could easily see how our prostates become diseased and how our lives can be negatively affected by conventional treatments for prostate problems.

So much depends on a healthy prostate and a healthy prostate depends so much on how we treat our bodies.

In Chapter 2, learn how men have been unknowingly increasing their chances of getting a prostate problem from a very early age.

Chapter 2: The Prostate Health Diet

Our food is the secret to our health and wellness **or** our sickness and misery. Food, in its broadest definition of your daily inputs, is the single most important determinant of your health and your prostate's condition. It can cause us to sink or rise in health little by little.

This discourse will go beyond anything you have read elsewhere because, in all of my studies, I have never fully encountered the depth of what I offer to you in this book: the perfect diet for you and your prostate!

The Prostate Health Diet is not a one-size fits all diet. This diet puts the focus on you and your specific needs.

It is important to realize that there is diet theory and then there is reality. I have followed expert pundit advice, and it often made my health condition worse.

Every book I have read on health and diet, and every practitioner I have met, all seem to have very specific ideas about what constitutes the ideal diet.

It's easy to get stuck thinking that the foods you eat—or the diet you are on—are the best. You've studied it, adopted it and have a lot invested in your choice, habits and opinion.

Hey, I know! I did that for 35 years following a well-known pundit's advice! I just **knew** mine was the best until one night I woke up and could not pee at all! After that I followed other experts.

I worked from home where the quality of air, water and food was excellent and where I could easily implement health regimes without having to compromise. You could say I was the perfect candidate to test the various diets.

But my prostate only seemed to get worse! There certainly were good elements in their diet plans, so why in the world did I get worse instead of better?

Sometimes out of the blue I would have a sudden shut down strike me in the middle of the night. I couldn't urinate no matter how badly I had to!

I started to learn that certain deviations or indulgences (which were very rare, let me tell you!) could be very costly to the health of my prostate, so I avoided them as much as I could.

I then learned two things that provided a huge breakthrough:

- how to personally test to know if something I was going to eat would be good for me or not and
- how to avoid or prepare many common natural foods to minimize a relatively unknown harmful anti-nutrient that was weakening me and causing an almost allergic reaction.

These new breakthroughs were so profound that they started a shift in my health and—at long last—I began to recover.

For most of us, change is not easy because we get comfortable in our ways. But in the case of your prostate condition, the benefits of being pain free and healthy are well worth the effort to change.

The Prostate Health Diet is your perfect diet, customized for you by you, dynamically evolving in real-time and based on key principles that will make complete sense to you.

Look at some of the potential rewards of your prostate health diet:

- Avoid the risk of some serious side effects from conventional medical options like incontinence and impotence. I don't know about you but these two alone were enough to motivate me!
- Improve your overall health and wellbeing, which can add years to your life and life to your years with fewer "what ails ya?" as you age.
- Feel and look younger.
- Lose weight and feel great!
- Save money, if you have to pay for conventional healthcare. Avoiding costly procedures can be a significant savings in both money and time.

I am now going to share what I believe will be the answer to set you on the road to health.

You Are The Cause!

First, a prostate problem in your life means that you are doing some-thing harmful to your body. Disease does not mysteriously arise without causes.

This insight should be the basis of all medical practice, but sadly it is not. Western conventional medical practice only sees the condition or symptom. That is why it is known as symptomatic medicine. The Western approach fails to truly find the causes in order to change or cure the condition and allow healing to happen at the deepest level.

Without finding the causes and treating the symptoms, you are often left with unpleasant side effects and the recurrence of the problem later or a manifestation in another area of the body. The conditions that caused the problem in the first place have not been changed.

We evolved over thousands of years based on eating **real** food, not the artificial manufactured food that dominates our diets today.

Is it possible for today's foods to be healthy when they contain chemical ingredients that we cannot even pronounce? Can foods grown in soil containing artificial fertilizers and doused with pesticides and herbicides really be health enhancing?

You know the answers!

Over time—sometimes decades—those toxins work their way through our bodies and can eventually cause serious chronic disease. Chronic disease is the outcome of the body's last-ditch effort to isolate the toxins to protect itself to survive the onslaught.

As a result, prostate disease is now epidemic in the West. Your prostate sits between two organs of elimination: the bladder and the colon. The more toxic your diet, the more toxic your urine and feces are. Your prostate is vulnerable to absorbing these toxins.

In fact, your urine passes right through your prostate on its way out, and your rectum is adjacent to your prostate, separated by only the thin rectal wall. That is why a trained urologist can feel the condition of your prostate, whether you have an enlarged or cancerous one, by the infamous digital rectal exam.

The slow development of prostate disease is why men often face prostate ailments at midlife: enlargement, infection and cancers.

Prevention is so much easier than reversing the damage. **Proper prostate nutrition is crucial**. It is never too early to start or too late to reap the benefits. The first step is to stop eating toxic food. The next step is to start eating healthy foods.

What's The Best Diet For You?

Isn't that the key question?

To answer it, I must ask you to decide the following:

1. Are you willing to do the work? Or do you want results without effort and commitment?

2. Are you seduced by wild promises that mean nothing in the end but disappointment? Have you been there before?

3. Are you willing to suspend your beliefs to learn something new?

If you feel a YES inside you to the above answers, let's begin . . .

Everyone is unique. Our nutritional needs vary based on our genetic inheritance or constitution, our health condition at the present time, and the toxic footprint we have added to our bodies over a lifetime.

The ratios of nutrients from foods—carbohydrates, proteins and fats as well as the need for different vitamins and minerals—vary from person to person.

If a diet does not address our individuality—our biochemical uniqueness and health condition—then it is not the answer. It may work for a select few.

There are some basic things to consider before you start tailoring the diet for you and your body. Let's take a look at those first.

How the 20ᵗʰ Century Changed the West's Food

During the 20th century, the West's agricultural practices changed dramatically and have seen huge increases in the following:

- hormones fed to animals
- contaminants and chemicals in our water supplies
- using grains, an unnatural primary food for cows, as the main input to increase milk and meat production with unhealthy consequences for them and us
- pasteurization and homogenization of milk and dairy products
- chemicalized production of vegetable oils
- consumption of denatured grains like white breads, cakes and cookies
- consumption of trans fats and hardened fats like margarine
- sugar consumption, as well as deadly artificial sugar consumption
- excessive medications of all kinds
- harmful vaccines
- fluoridation and chlorination of our water supplies
- regular feeding of animal by-products to livestock
- bioconcentration of toxins up the food chain
- chemical fertilizer use, herbicides and pesticides
- factory farms in which animals are confined to tiny spaces and are kept from developing severe diseases only by extensive antibiotic use
- using city sewage (sludge) for farms as fertilizer with concentrations of residues and toxins from all kinds of manufactured products and medical discards
- the use of only a few seed types, which diminishes our variety and the trace elements found in a diverse food supply
- monoculture crop methods over the last century that depletes the mineral content of the soil, as this farming method relies on petroleum-based chemical fertilizers that deplete soil of vital minerals, including zinc and selenium, both of which are crucial to prostate health
- genetically modified (GM) foods, something that is so alien and unknown to our bodies, are now found in almost all soy, sugar beet and corn products that make up the bulk of our fast foods and supermarket foods (and many commercial supplement ingredients)

All of these changes impact the quality of our food, denature it and lead to disease, especially when combined with other Western lifestyle choices.

Time is the critical factor here. While one meal will not have a high impact or effect, decades of these types of foods will ultimately lead to chronic disease, which is now considered epidemic in the West.

Food Manufacturing Practices

The above list of recent changes to agricultural approaches does not include the food manufacturing practices, which are even more toxic:

- adding high fructose corn syrup in most prepared foods and soft drinks
- using artificial sweeteners that are alien to the body and not metabolized properly

- using MSG and its derivatives like hydrolyzed protein, which are carcinogenic
- adding all kinds of toxic preservatives and chemicals to our food
- stripping nutrients from our grain products by removing the hulls and more to make them "white"
- drastically increasing the sugar and salt content in our food
- adding artificial flavorings and colorings
- using chemicals and high heat in manufacturing vegetable oils
- using margarine and trans fats in food preparation

To read more about harmful ingredients found commonly in supermarket foods, read the article: *What's Really in the Food?* (tiny.cc/v9xrzw)

You know all these things! You may have been relying on a strong constitution to temporarily avoid disaster or have bought into the medical symptomatic view of the world that disease just "happens."

As I have said before, you can change this. Disease is not inevitable.

Slowly Toxins Become Your Enemy

The toxic overload of estrogen-mimicking and hormone-disrupting chemicals (known as "xenoestrogens)—in our soil, in our food, in the air, in the water, in our personal care and household products—alters our hormone balance and leads to prostate problems.

It is no wonder we suffer so many ailments!

Hormone disruptors are the pesticides, herbicides and fungicides associated with non-organic food, the chemicals that are leached into food from food-can linings and water from plastic bottles, the cleaners you use in your house and the non-stick surfaces in your pots and pans, the fireproofed mattresses and synthetic clothing.

Men now have extremely high levels of estrogen, which causes changes in men's testosterone levels and, therefore, male breast growth, erectile difficulties and lower sperm count—never mind obesity. Men are almost guaranteed to have some form of prostate disease—including prostate cancer—as they age unless they stop the prime causes.

We consume so many foods laced with chemicals and xenoestrogens that our bodies are fighting to survive. To me, it is no mystery why we have such sky-high rates of prostate conditions.

It reminds me of the story of the frog in a pot of water. Heat it slowly and the frog stays until boiled to death!

How to stop the causes? **Minimize** the inputs of toxicity and **maximize** cleansing and high quality food inputs. You can reverse the damages done over the decades or at least minimize the severity of disease. Men's prostate health requires optimal natural food choices.

BPA

Bisphenol A is found in the lining of the cans your canned food comes in and in some plastics used for water. Just like that, you have an even greater burden of toxins!

BPA is an endocrine disruptor that mimics estrogen. It is linked to imbalanced hormone levels and decreased testosterone. Just what your prostate needs, right?

If we add toxins in our diet—whether knowingly or not—we automatically stress our prostate and deposit toxins into it. Lo and behold, one day prostate disease strikes, seemingly out of the blue. Well, now you know the real cause, and the solution is obvious: change your inputs!

Neurotoxins

Neurotoxins are added to many manufactured and restaurant foods as taste enhancers. This is true of many healthy sounding chemicals, including many organic ones.

These ingredients often cause serious health reactions over time, adding to the body's toxic load, and cause food addictions and weight gain. We need to educate ourselves to read labels. There are just too many deadly, manufactured additives hidden in packaged and restaurant food, such as MSG.

> *Monosodium glutamate (MSG) is probably the best known of the neuro-toxins. However, there are many other names for these protein additives . . . Even the pleasant sounding term "natural flavors" can mean the presence of additives toxic to the brain and nervous system . . .*
>
> *When the word "spices" is used, it is the tip-off that toxic additives are hidden in the product . . . There is no way to know unless you are willing to take the time to read the label."*
>
> *A Hundred Health Sapping Neurotoxins are Hidden in Packaged and Restaurant Food by B. L. Minton,* tiny.cc/mcyrzw

Here are some other neurotoxic chemical food additives:

- aspartame Nutrasweet
- beef flavoring
- protein concentrate
- bouillon protein extract
- caseinate seasoned salt
- chicken flavoring seasoning
- smoke flavoring
- glutamate soy extract
- hydrolyzed ingredients
- soy protein
- corn protein
- wheat protein
- milk solids spice
- monosodium glutamate

- textured vegetable protein
- natural flavor
- yeast extract

The best thing you can do is start reading your labels **before** buying your food!

Pesticides

The pesticides in our food are powerful endocrine disruptors. They directly affect our hormones. In the case of men, pesticides in our food result in excess female estrogens and weaken the prostate gland that relies on healthy levels of testosterone to be in optimum shape.

Pesticides also affect body weight and mood, increase your risk of prostate cancer and lower your sperm count. No wonder so many couples cannot conceive naturally today!

Most Americans eat over a gallon of pesticides and health-destroying chemicals each year! Although many of these toxic chemicals are excreted, our immune system eventually becomes compromised. Our fat tissues absorb these toxins and, in many cases, cause weight gain and the onset of chronic health conditions.

We know the enemy now—from government to agribiz to mass processed food manufacturers, from fast food chains to our supermarkets and restaurants—and finally us who consumes them! We are our own worst enemy!

The Environmental Working Group (EWG) studied the amount of residues of pesticides found on 47 fruits and vegetables, and 87,000 tests were made between 2000 and 2007, leading to a classification of the most to the least contaminated and toxic produce. Read more on pesticides applied to produce in *EWG's Shopper's Guide*: www.ewg.org/foodnews/

Here is a list of the worst pesticide foods—the higher the number, the worse the food:

peach	100	green beans	53
apple	93	summer squash	53
sweet bell pepper	83	pepper	51
celery	82	cucumber	50
nectarine	81	raspberries	46
strawberries	80	grapes (domestic)	44
cherries	73	plums	44
kale	69	oranges	44
lettuce	67	cauliflower	39
grapes (imported)	66	tangerines	37
carrots	63	mushrooms	36
pear	63	bananas	34
collard greens	60	winter squash	34
spinach	58	cantaloupe	33
potatoes	56		

cranberries	33	kiwi	13
honeydew melon	30	sweet peas (frozen)	10
grapefruit	29	asparagus	10
sweet potatoes	29	mango	9
tomatoes	29	pineapple	7
broccoli	28	sweet corn (frozen)	2
watermelon	26	avocado	1
papaya	20	onion	1
eggplant	20		
cabbage	17		

Note. 100 = worst pesticide load; 1 = least pesticide load.

It is in your best interest to switch to organic versions of anything over 25. The others you could get away with if need be, but the food would still lack optimum nutrient density because of the depleted soils they were grown in. Non-organic produce may look great, but it is deficient in selenium and a host of other minerals essential for your health.

Genetically Modified Foods

Countries around the world are banning genetically modified and genetically engineered foods. The American Academy of Environmental Medicine has issued a warning to avoid genetically modified foods, which you can read about at the following link, and come to your own conclusions (tiny.cc/rfyrzw).

Nobody knows the consequences of splicing in new genes and eating that product for several generations. What is known is that when GMO's flooded the market, food related illnesses DOUBLED. GMO foods can be:

- Allergenic
- Toxic
- Carcinogenic
- Anti-nutritional

Plus, GM crops are grown with the herbicide Roundup, which has been linked to numerous physiological problems in humans, including birth defects and the destruction of testosterone and male fertility (tiny.cc/xiyrzw).

Dr. Mercola gives an amazing comparison of the nutritional value of GM corn versus non-GM corn:

> *Genetic modification is also making our modern food less nutritious than it used to be, according to a report given to MomsAcrossAmerica by an employee of De Dell Seed Company (Canada's only non-GMO corn seed company). It offers a stunning picture of the nutritional differences between genetically modified (GM) and non-GM corn. Clearly, the former is NOT equivalent to the latter, which is the very premise by which genetically modified crops were approved in the first place. Here's a small sampling of the nutritional differences found in this 2012 nutritional analysis:*
>
> - *Calcium: GMO corn = 14 ppm/Non-GMO corn = 6,130 ppm (437 times more)*

- *Magnesium: GMO corn = 2 ppm/Non-GMO corn = 113 ppm (56 times more)*
- *Manganese: GMO corn = 2 ppm/Non-GMO corn = 14 ppm (7 times more)*

Breeding the Nutrition Out of Our Food by Dr. Mercola, tiny.cc/sjyrzw

For an in-depth education on the many dangers of GM foods, Jeffrey Smith's books document at least 65 serious health risks from GM products of all kinds—*Seeds of Deception: Exposing Industry and Government Lies About the Safety of the Genetically Engineered Foods You're Eating* (tiny.cc/hlyrzw).

For more, read these articles: *Roundup and Birth Defects: Is the Public Being Kept in the Dark?* (tiny.cc/jmyrzw) and *Study: Roundup Diluted by 99.8 percent Still Destroys Human DNA* (tiny.cc/ioyrzw).

To know more about the effects on animal livers and kidneys, visit this site: tiny.cc/ypyrzw

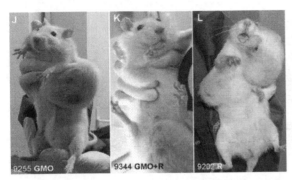

Reprinted from Food and Chemical Toxicology, 50(11), Séralini, G., Clair E., Mesnage, R., Gress, S., Defarge, N., Malatesta, M., Hennequin, D., & de Vendômois, J. S. *Long Term Toxicity of a Roundup Pesticide and a Roundup-tolerant Genetically Modified Maize.* Copyright (2012), with permission from Elsevier. tiny.cc/c2yrzw

A 2009 Brazilian study published findings about significant changes in rat uteruses and reproductive cycles: *The Anatomical Record* (tiny.cc/nyyrzw). Another 2009 French study, published in the *International Journal of Biological Sciences*, revealed the long-term effects on rats of Monsanto corn with trace amounts of the chemical fertilizer, Roundup (tiny.cc/5zyrzw). The lab rats developed grotesque tumours, organ damage and premature death.

Read more about Irina Ermakova's study on mother rats fed GM soy at the Russian National Academy of Sciences, *GM Soy Dangerous to Newborns?* tiny.cc/c2yrzw

Many countries around the world are banning GMO foods.

Avoid processed foods, which are certain to contain up to 70% GM foods. Corn and soy are in the vast majority of all processed and fast food products!

Download the *Non-GMO Shopping Guide*, issued by the Institute for Responsible Technology at www.nongmoshoppingguide.com/

Vitamins & Minerals

In Chapter 8, I go into great lengths about how to get the vitamins and minerals from food sources and when to supplement in pill form, which should be done at a minimum. What I want to talk about here is deficiency, depletion and anti-nutrients.

There is just not enough nutrition in the food we eat in the Standard American Diet (SAD). Traditional, time-tested methods of food preparation can ensure we get the minerals we need from our healthy, organic food. The bottom line is that vitamin and mineral deficiencies are another key cause of disease.

Depletion

Let's take a look at how depleted our food has become from our modern commercial farming practices. This short list from the U.S. Department of Agriculture indicates the nutritional values for fruits and vegetables versus what they were in 1975:

Fruit or Vegetable	Nutritional Value Change since 1975
Apples	Vitamin A is down 41%
Sweet Peppers	Vitamin C is down 31%
Watercress	Iron is down 88%
Broccoli	Calcium and Vitamin A are down 50%
Cauliflower	Vitamin C is down 45%; Vitamin B1 is down 48%; Vitamin B2 is down 47%
Collards Greens	Vitamin A is down 45%; Potassium is down 60%; Magnesium is down 85%

Wow! Our food has been designed to look good and store well in transit to supermarkets, but the vitamin and mineral content of our food has dramatically plummeted.

Deficiency

Eating conventional foods is a quick way to rob your body of essential nutrients! No wonder organic foods have been growing at a compound rate of 25% per year for well over a decade. Many consumers have realized that the price of conventional food is sky high in terms of its deleterious effect on our health.

> *Trace minerals like zinc and selenium are absolutely crucial to the proper functioning of your body. And yet, nearly all trace minerals are widely depleted in the soils that grow our food.*
>
> *That's because conventional agriculture extracts these minerals from the soils, year after year, while replenishing none of them. Conventional fertilizers contain virtually no trace minerals, so after just one decade of growing crops through conventional methods, the soils are depleted of crucial trace minerals that your body needs to function. Conventional agriculture, it turns out, is almost like a strip mining operation that pulls valuable minerals out of the soil and carries them away in the food, ultimately leaving the soils depleted.*
>
> *Why You Should Get Your Selenium and Zinc from Foods, Not Synthetic Vitamins by M. Adams, tiny.cc/38yrzw*

If you think just taking a mineral supplement solves that problem, you have been misinformed as this book will show you.

Anti-Nutrients

An anti-nutrient is a natural or synthetic compound that interferes with your body's absorption of vitamins, minerals or other nutrients. Perhaps the most important one for prostate health is phytic acid.

What is Phytic Acid?

A wide range of food types contain the anti-nutrient phytic acid, otherwise known as phytates. Phytic acid occurs naturally in whole grains, beans, pulses, nuts and seeds to help these plants defend against their insect predators and prevent premature germination thereby making it possible for them to be stored for a long time.

Phytic acid acts as an irritant in the human body while gradually removing vital minerals over time as you eat foods that contain it, unless they are prepared properly in time-tested traditional ways. **Phytic acid binds with calcium, iron, zinc and magnesium, and it removes them from the body**.

These minerals are especially important for vibrant health, a lack of which can cause all sorts of health problems that seem to materialize later in life. Cumulative reductions in these elements over time take their toll.

In the particular case of the male reproductive system, zinc deficiencies are a real problem because the prostate requires lots of zinc to function properly.

"Zinc deficiency can lead to numerous health conditions, including prostate disorders which may in turn lead to prostate cancer." Read the article *Zinc is Essential for Good Health* (tiny.cc/jazrzw).

The reduction in calcium levels also helps produce cavities and osteoporosis. Combined with low levels of magnesium, you have a recipe for many diseases. For more information, see *Magnesium is Vital for Good Health* (tiny.cc/hbzrzw).

Magnesium is an absolute necessity within our bodies, especially these days when our intake of and exposure to toxins and heavy metals is so high and occurs on a daily basis. With accumulation of toxins and acid residues, our bodies will degenerate and age more quickly. Simply put, magnesium is needed for the survival of our cells.

A deficiency of this mineral sets the stage for cancer. It's an extremely powerful mineral with the ability to rejuvenate and prevent calcification of organs and tissues.

More and more research is showing the benefits of magnesium both as a method of detoxing the body from heavy metals built up over time in the body and as a key element in the natural treatment of cancer. Most of us can use additions of magnesium. The best way to increase your magnesium intake is with a simple water-based spray applied to the skin—a very inexpensive and effective mineral to use.

> *Magnesium does protect cells from aluminum, mercury, lead, cadmium, beryllium and nickel, which explains why re-mineralization is so essential for heavy metal detoxification and chelation as well as radiation protection. Magnesium is essential for the survival of our cells but takes on further importance now where our bodies are being bombarded on a daily basis with heavy metals and radiation.*

Magnesium Offers Strong Radiation Protection by M. Sircus, tiny.cc/pczrzw

For more information on the benefits of magnesium, visit Dr. Sircus' Blog—Magnesium Oil site (drsircus.com/medicine/magnesium). Foods high in magnesium include beans (black and kidney), green vegetables (broccoli and spinach), seafood (oysters, rockfish, halibut and scallops), nuts and seeds (sesame, flax, almonds, cashews, pumpkin and squash seeds), lentils, bran (rice, oats and wheat), cacao, molasses and herbs.

Another detriment of phytates in foods is its deleterious effect on digestion, causing all kinds of problems. Phytic acid inhibits enzymes needed for digestion including pepsin for breaking down proteins in the stomach, amylase for turning starch into sugar and trypsin needed for digesting protein in the small intestine.

You can download a comprehensive article about phytates here: *Cereal Grains: Humanity's Double-Edged Sword* (tiny.cc/wfzrzw).

For another thorough article on phytic acid and reduction techniques, please read this article: *Living with Phytic Acid* (tiny.cc/sgzrzw).

Phytic Acid Levels in Some Foods

The following is a list of foods containing the anti-nutrient phytic acid (phytates). It is not that we should stop eating these food groups, but rather we must learn how to remove phytates through proper, traditional methods of food preparation. Otherwise we risk unexplained disease development over time.

Soaking or fermenting are the primary ways of reducing phytates, while sprouting and sourdough leavening help. If phytate-rich foods are not soaked first, the phytates remain in the food.

One of the worst offenders are cereal flakes and puffed grains. The high-heat extrusion process exaggerates the phytates, which makes these supposed healthy cereals into deadly culprits! For more information, read the article *Eating Cardboard is 'Healthier' than Breakfast Cereal* (tiny.cc/tjzrzw)

As a wise preventative measure, start changing your cooking habits with these foods:

Food	Phytic Acid (mg/100g)
Sesame seeds dehulled	5,360
100% Wheat bran cereal	3,290
Soybeans	1,000–2,220
Cocoa powder	1,684–1,796
Oats	1,370
Brown rice	1,250
Oat flakes	1,174
Coconut meal	1,170
Almonds	1,138–1,400
Parboiled brown rice	1,600
Barley	1,190

Food	Phytic Acid (mg/100g)
Whole corn	1,050
Rye	1,010
Walnut	982
Whole wheat flour	960
Lentils	779
Navy beans	740–1,780
Hazelnuts	648–1,000
Wild rice flour	634–753
Refried beans	622
Peanuts germinated	610
Pinto beans	600–2,380
Corn tortillas	448
Corn	367
White flour	258
White flour tortillas	123

Note. Measurements are in milligrams per 100 grams of weight. *Source*: (Part I) Whole Grain Toxicity—Phytic Acid Contained in Popular Foods, tiny.cc/umzrzw

The Weston A. Price Foundation documents:

> *What researchers often overlook is the fact that seed foods—grains, legumes and nuts—are prepared with great care in traditional societies, by sprouting, roasting, soaking, fermenting and sour leavening. These processes neutralize substances in whole grains and other seed foods that block mineral absorption, inhibit protein digestion and irritate the lining of the digestive tract. Such processes also increase nutrient content and render seed foods more digestible.*
>
> *Nasty, Brutish and Short?* by S. F. Morell, tiny.cc/8ozrzw

To learn more about phytates and to get great recipes, read: *Rebuild Market—Phytic Acid Drill-Down* (tiny.cc/4qzrzw).

These phytate-rich foods, unless prepared properly, can trigger unexplained sudden prostate attacks (e.g., blockages, very frequent urination and more). I believe that phytates are a big part of why we have enlarged prostates and other prostate diseases, especially when coupled with our many poor diet habits and with depleted, commercial toxic foods.

I HIGHLY recommend reading a book called *Nourishing Traditions: The Cookbook that Challenges Politically Correct Nutrition and the Diet Dictocrats* (tiny.cc/3tzrzw). Despite its title, this book will educate you on the whys and hows of proper food preparation. It is a fantastic book filled with all kinds of great mouth-watering recipes, dietary information and important phytate-reducing techniques.

Please do get the book if a lot of what I say is new to you and if you need help in how to prepare your meals. Tons of superb recipes!

Here is another great source of info and tips: *Phytic Acid—Tips for Consumers from Food Science* (www.phyticacid.org/)

Here is another detailed explanation of phytic acid in foods. While the source is from a Paleo diet perspective, about which I have some reservations as described later, this is an excellent insight into some dangers in supposedly healthy food choices. See *What's Wrong with Beans and Legumes*, tiny.cc/l0zrzw

Once I started personal testing (see Chapter 9), I realized how wrong I was when I assumed that my prior long-time vegan diet of grains, nuts, seeds and vegetables was perfect for me. Now I know what triggered such severe reactions in my prostate: anti-nutrients like phytic acid! It was humbling for me to admit that I had been wrong for 35 years! I needed to challenge my past assumptions and really examine what foods were ideal for me in each moment. It was also empowering to find the answers at long last to heal my prostate condition!

Prepare Your Food with Traditional, Time-Tested Methods

If you are very healthy, small daily amounts of phytate-rich foods may not be harmful as your body can deal with them, while sensitive constitutions will have reactions. However, large amounts over time are a recipe for severe health problems.

Fortunately, there are ways of preparing your grains, beans, pulses, nuts and seeds that reduce the level of phytic acid.

The first step is to soak foods that have anti-nutrients to reduce their harmful effect on the body. Then you can either sprout them or cook them with some sea salt to further reduce the remaining phytates.

This is a highly useful chart for that purpose. Just drag it onto your desktop and then print it out: *The Whole Food Lab Soak & Sprout* at www.wholefoodlab.com/soak-sprout/.

Nuts are easy to soak. In lukewarm water, dissolve some sea salt and soak the nuts overnight. Then rinse and dry at around 150°F until crunchy. I use my toaster oven for that.

For grains, soak overnight or first thing in the morning for supper. Rinse and cook. By the way, soaked foods will cook much faster.

Beans are best to soak longer (12–24 hours) and start with warm water. Rinse and cook. Adding some kombu seaweed also will help digestion. These steps allow not only for reduction of the harmful elements but also improve absorption of the minerals and nutrients by your body.

Eat According to Your Local Climate

Eat according to your environment, climate and season. When you do, your body adjusts properly to your climate by releasing the right amount of vitamin D, which ensures proper digestion.

Although we can eat out-of-season foods due to modern conveniences of transport and cooling, eating foods regularly from other climates and zones will shut down your proper digestion and wreak havoc with your hormones—and that is the last thing you want to do for your prostate!

Eat local, which puts you in the correct zone in the right season. Get sun on your skin. If you can't get sun, then minimize raw food and cut out tropical foods. Why? Because sun tells your body that in-season raw food is fine to eat.

If you ignore your climate and the foods that are ideal for you there, you will be inputting foods that will compromise your health over time.

Raw foods may be great for a short time in a hot climate, but imagine eating bananas and watermelons regularly in Alaska in the middle of a deep freeze in January! Sure, as a treat, you will be fine, but as part of a long-term diet of raw vegetables, fruits, etc., you will eventually damage your body.

Sounds drastic, doesn't it? But once you know about the ileocecal valve, all of this makes sense. Your ileocecal valve is located between the large and small intestine. It keeps the flora in your large intestine from backing up into the small intestine where it can wreak havoc.

Eating the wrong foods in the wrong climate at the wrong time of year weakens your ileocecal valve so that it doesn't close properly. To stay strong, this valve needs calcium, magnesium and vitamin D produced in your body.

But your body won't produce vitamin D if you are eating foods from other parts of the world and foods that are out of season. All plant-derived foods contain potassium. Tropical plant-based foods have higher levels of potassium. When we eat them, our kidneys register the higher levels of potassium and, as if they could think, assume we are in a sunny location and getting a lot of sun and vitamin D. Therefore, the body doesn't need to produce vitamin D. Ooops!

All of a sudden, you'll have difficulty with proper digestion. You might not notice this—it depends on many other factors. When there is trouble digesting, watch out! Your liver then becomes burdened with bad bacteria, which creates further havoc with your digestion and, in time, with your health. This results in food reactions, irritable bowel and a host of problems for your prostate including the inability to deploy hormones properly.

Dr. Jonn Matsen, an amazing world class Naturopathic Doctor, has written a truly insightful book on the wide range of chronic health problems that plague modern society.

The simple message he says is this:

> *If you're not actually out in the sun, you could quickly lose your calcium absorption—and within five days, your ileocecal valve could be weak enough to allow your billions of good bacteria to stampede into your small intestine, where they could become Bad Guys.*
>
> *The Yeast Are Back by J. Matsen,* tiny.cc/q6zrzw

So, eating the highest quality food, if not attuned to your climate and season, can actually worsen your condition or delay your healing! This is **really important** to keep in mind!

His solution is to stop eating raw food for six days. Add high quality sea salt to your lightly cooked vegetables. Take a high quality vitamin D and the Cal Mag liquid supplement that he recommends (tiny.cc/ca0rzw) as well as and the SC Liver Formula (tiny.cc/eb0rzw).

Take the 6 day test as above, and you will see the difference it makes. YOU WILL BE AMAZED! I was.

Then you can start on his program of killing off the yeast overgrowth. We all have yeast in the large intestine—sometimes too much—and you will be stunned at the difference it makes to your health!

Bio-Nutritional Formulas—Latero Flora Powder (tiny.cc/ze0rzw)

It is best to start with 1/8th of a teaspoon every 3 days and then increase to a 1/4 teaspoon. You do not want to rush the yeast kill as it is too hard on your liver when that happens too fast. So adjust accordingly and start slow.

Read more in his book, which easily explains what ails you and why it is happening. The book is filled with simple cartoon diagrams that simplify complex issues so they are easy to understand.

He has seen tens of thousands of patients and has had stunning results. He's known for "curing the incurable." He is a very affordable, warm and friendly doctor.

His discourse on the dangers of amalgam fillings is world class as are his perspectives on vaccines.

I highly recommend you read this book, *Eating Alive II*, especially if you have mercury fillings or if you are not making progress in your healing (tiny.cc/1g0rzw).

This unseasonal, non-local eating is one of the causes of long-term chronic health conditions and weight gain. Without optimum digestion, you are doomed to many side effects, some minor and some major.

Cooked vegetables are easier to digest than raw foods, especially in the winter in colder climates. Eat local and eat smart! You can easily test this by seeing which response is stronger when you personally test: cooked or raw foods of the same type. Read Chapter 9 to learn more about personal testing.

Now read on to learn more about vitamin D and sunlight.

Sunlight Exposure

Not enough sunlight—this is a leading cause of prostate cancer. In northerly climates, there are fewer sunlight hours and more exposure is needed. Vitamin D, the single most important nutrient for good health, actually acts like a hormone in the body.

Vitamin D studies show that most people today are deficient in this essential vitamin and that increased amounts of vitamin D in your body reduces your cancer risk by 50% or more, including prostate cancer!

Most modern Western men are terribly low in vitamin D, especially black or darker-skinned Americans, whose skin color was designed to withstand lots of daily sun exposure. Black Americans have the highest rates of prostate cancer. Many practitioners correlate that risk with low levels of vitamin D.

In the winter in the U.S., most people are extremely deficient in vitamin D because of the lack of sun exposure. Even people who live in sunny climates, but spend too much time indoors, can be very deficient, too.

We have been sold on the fact that sun exposure is bad for us. Now people avoid the sun completely, cover up when out or use chemical sunscreens, which are actually toxic and cancer causing.

Overwhelming evidence indicates that people benefit from sun exposure. Responsible sun exposure, which means avoiding the strongest midday rays, is so beneficial and needs to be done **without** sunscreen for at least 15–20 minutes per day. This is by far the best supplement of all!

If you have sensitive skin, build up slowly with just a few minutes and then augment until you get at least 20 minutes over as much of your body surface as possible, ideally including the prostate area. There is something to say for nudist colonies!

The darker your skin is naturally, the longer this daily exposure should be (i.e., over 20 minutes) as it takes longer to absorb the needed amount of vitamin D. If you want to use a sunscreen during midday, use an *Organic Zinc Oxide Sunscreen* (tiny.cc/cj0rzw).

"Vitamin D is the single most effective medicine against cancer, far outpacing the benefits of any cancer drug known to modern science." *New Research Shows Vitamin D Slashes Risk of Cancers by 77 Percent: Cancer Industry Refuses to Support Cancer Prevention* (tiny.cc/yk0rzw).

I urge you to become better informed about sun exposure because it is such an important issue for your health. Here are several good sources of information regarding sunlight and vitamin D:

"Vitamin D is the single most effective medicine against cancer, far outpacing the benefits of any cancer drug known to modern science." *The Healing Benefits of Sunlight and Vitamin D* (tiny.cc/8l0rzw)

The Sunscreen Myth: How Sunscreen Products Actually Promote Cancer (tiny.cc/gn0rzw)

7 Surprising Things You're Not Supposed to Know about Sunscreen and Sunlight Exposure (tiny.cc/ko0rzw)

"Epidemic" of Vitamin D Deficiency: MUHC study (tiny.cc/f64wzw)

Higher Vitamin D Intake Needed to Reduce Cancer Risk (tiny.cc/874wzw)

If you are not already convinced, read the comprehensive information provided by the Vitamin D Council (www.vitamindcouncil.org/).

If you can't get sun exposure due to dark, cloudy days—or because you lack the time—then the best way to supplement is with sardines or potent cod liver oil (see *Cod Liver Oil* in Chapter 8). This way you are getting your vitamin D direct from a food source rather than a manufactured supplement.

The next best choice for vitamin D is natural vitamin D3 supplements, but this is nowhere near as good as the cod liver oil, which has been time tested over thousands of years. See *Vitamin D* in Chapter 8.

Exercise

Any writer who talks about good health and diet has to urge readers to take up exercise as a key component of turning your health around or of maintaining the gifts of good health.

If you want to lose weight then no matter how well you eat, you cannot get full mileage out of your diet without revving up the metabolic engine.

Exercise is essential to add quality and length to your life. Our sedentary lifestyles impact our prostates directly. It is crucial to add movement throughout the day to counteract the effects of so much sitting time, and your prostate will be happy!

We were born to move our bodies every day. We all know that we need to add exercising into our daily routines for weight and health benefits.

I will share some tips with you that I have gleaned over the years of doing these sports: running including 3 marathons; swimming; biking; hiking and mountaineering; climbing; skiing—all types, especially back-country telemarking; ultimate Frisbee (football with a Frisbee); yoga and tai chi.

Tips

- Do something you love.
- You can get in shape for a sport by doing body exercises (that use your own weight rather than dumb dumbbells): push ups and pull ups, squats and lunges, or skipping.
- Learning how to breathe properly while moving is extremely important. Breathe in and out through your nose, not your mouth. Make the out-breath powerful by pulling your stomach in at the same time.
- Training with bursts of intensity is far more beneficial than steady pacing, and it saves a lot of time—10 minutes will do you!
- Do 10–30 second bursts of high intensity exercise at your level. If you start out with walking, then after warming up for a bit, walk as fast as you can for 10 seconds

followed by 1–2 minutes of slow walking while your breath and heartbeat return to normal. Then repeat several more times. Work your way up to 30 second bursts. Same for running or swimming.

- Varying routines prevents injuries.
- Stretching also helps avoid injury.
- By doing something you love, exercising becomes enjoyable rather than a burden.

Conclusion

Modern factory-manufactured food, toxicity, vitamin and mineral deficiencies and lack of sunshine are the main reasons men have prostate problems.

It is time to get back to our roots. Simpler food and healthier lifestyles have to become the priority in day-to-day living, not an afterthought.

Real food costs more . . . but in the end, it saves you money and just may save you! Many consumers have realized that the price of conventional food is sky high in terms of its deleterious effect on their health.

The answer is clear: food can be your medicine or your poison.

If you want food to be your medicine, read on. Chapter 3 gives you a clear idea of changes you can make to your diet.

Chapter 3: Levels of Healthy Eating

In this section, I provide a scale of the poorest diet to the most ideal—or optimum—diet. This scale offers a benchmark to test where your diet ranks and a clear path for how to begin changing your diet, step by step.

Most people believe they eat a healthy diet. If this is true, then why do we have an epidemic of prostate diseases and such a poor quality of life as we age?

Why are so many elderly people excessively unhealthy and reliant on drugs? Why are we not vital until old age like the Okinawans of Japan who work outdoors and live to a very old age and who have none of the awful health problems of most of our elderly?

Prostate diseases are rare in cultures that eat traditional natural foods. The medical profession would have you believe that poor prostate health results from the fact that we live longer. In truth, the accumulation of toxins from our modern, devitalized "non-foods," manufactured food concoctions and poor food preparation methods are the cause.

In your quest for healthier eating, you may encounter many so-called food experts who claim that their diet is what you need. My message over and over is nobody knows what's best for you—only you do.

A diet may recommend foods that may be harmful for one body, and there may be healthy foods that the diet says you should never touch that may be exactly what another body needs. It doesn't matter how much science is behind a diet—we are incredibly different from each other.

For example, many new diets come out of California, fad capital of the world! A raw diet that works well for someone in that hot sunny climate may be deadly for someone in a different climate. That's the problem with the diet gurus who claim their way is the best way.

The good news is that you can change from the diet you've been eating and find a new diet for your unique body. If you are transitioning from a chronic health condition, then most likely you will be highly sensitive or reactive to many foods. Don't despair! Once your condition and your health improve, you will be able to eat more widely with fewer—if any—reactions.

The following levels of healthy eating provide ideas so you can move up the levels and change your diet at a pace that works for you.

Poorest Diet

- artificial sweeteners of all kinds such as Aspartame (NutraSweet) and Splenda (Sucralose) and their products like diet soft drinks
- drinks and foods sweetened with fructose or high fructose corn syrup and its derivatives
- foods with preservatives, MSG and other hidden neurotoxic ingredients
- highly processed, manufactured factory foods
- foods containing growth hormones and antibiotics, like non-organic dairy and meats

- foods sprayed with pesticides
- GMO (Genetically Modified Organisms) foods, which are foreign to the body (90% of soy and corn and their products in the U.S. contain GMOs . . . and they are also fed to animals that you eat)
- food with vegetable trans fats
- commercial manufactured vegetable oils and margarines
- artificial food and food dyes
- meat from animals that are regularly fed grains not grasses—and animal parts—and are grown in animal factories, or a Concentrated Animal Feeding Operation (CAFO). More info at tiny.cc/ie6wzw
- BBQ'd food (burnt fat and charred meat are cancer causing)

Yikes! How in the world can we be healthy when we feed ourselves such non-foods? This is anything but a prostate health diet.

Poor Diet

- commercial sprayed crops (vegetables and fruit)
- refined carbs like white flours and sugars often laced with preservatives
- undetected molds in our food hidden by preservatives
- unripe fruit sprayed with pesticides
- commercial animal fat
- meat and fowl grown in cramped quarters, stuffed with antibiotics and fed low quality unnatural feed like grains instead of grasses and forage
- pasteurized and homogenized dairy food and milk
- high fructose corn syrup and its products
- desserts with unhealthy fats and sugar
- canned food in BPA-lined cans
- table salt
- microwaved food
- hydrogenated or partially hydrogenated oils and margarine
- processed or smoked meats, hot dogs, deli meats often containing preservatives
- commercial fast foods
- highly manufactured, packaged food with many ingredients
- boxed, puffed and flaked cereals; rice cakes; etc.

At best, you should only eat these foods rarely. Look at our epidemics of disease—from diabetes to heart ailments, from cancer to chronic illnesses, from overweight problems to degenerative diseases. Most commercial food and fast foods are highly responsible for these major health problems and diseases.

Acceptable Diet

- fresh food but no commercial meat, dairy or soy foods
- minimal processed and packaged supermarket foods
- minimal commercial vegetable oils and margarines, use butter/coconut oil instead
- home cooked meals using fresh ingredients
- free range fowl and meat

26

- frozen seafood
- no microwaved foods
- avoid GMO foods and ingredients
- restaurant food that isn't fast-food quality, that is made with GMO-free natural ingredients and that doesn't microwave food, if you can find such a restaurant

Good Food

- organic produce and dairy
- fresh seasonal local food
- fresh raw food
- seafood low on the scale of toxic metal fish
- free-range fowl and meat
- natural whole foods: grains, beans, seeds, nuts and produce
- sea salt
- organic restaurant food only

Optimum Food

- homegrown or locally farmed fresh organic fruits and vegetables
- organic wild berries
- real superfoods as part of the diet
- fresh organic raw food, sprouts (in moderation) and raw fermented vegetables
- balanced food for your particular body
- non-pasteurized organic dairy from grass-fed animals
- organic pasture grazed, grass-fed meat and fowl (not grain fed)
- fresh-caught seafood and shellfish lowest in toxic metal content
- organic whole foods: grains, beans, seeds and nuts soaked to reduce phytic acid and other anti-nutrients
- fresh wild foods and herbs

These lists shout out the differences based on our daily food choices. It can be a challenge to move up the scale, but it is a key choice if you want to prevent prostate problems.

In the long run, eating optimally will be the most important decision you can make for your health.

Food kills or food heals: it's your choice.

Conclusion

Food is very complex. Once you move up the scale then you want to be able to customize your diet for what really works for you, not based on theory. You need to know for sure that what you are eating is best for you.

The perfect diet for <u>you</u> is <u>not</u> for everyone! It doesn't matter what the food pundits, including me, claim. You are constantly changing and in need of different things from your food.

You are the master when it comes to knowing what is best for you to eat, but "knowing" requires learning, tuning inwards and listening to your body's needs. Your subconscious mind knows. In Chapter 9, I will provide you with a tool—called personal testing—that will help you to tune inwards and know what is good and what is bad for you **at this moment**. It is a simple and invaluable tool.

In Chapter 4, I review the most popular, contemporary diets, and you'll see why you must customize your diet for yourself.

Chapter 4: Popular Diets

I will examine many popular diets and explain their pros and cons, but before looking at specific diets, I want to look at two forms of diets that often get confused by many pundits: cleansing and nourishing diets.

Cleansing diets are used to eliminate toxins from the body, but are not ideal for long-term use. The reasons to use it should be to help accelerate the removal of debris and toxins that have accumulated in the organs and tissues of your body. Problems arise when we maintain a cleansing diet for too long.

These types of diets trigger a powerful immune response in the body which helps eliminate the bad stuff. If carried on for too long, our bodies get stressed and new types of problems develop. Always know if what you are doing is a cleansing program and remember that it has diminishing returns and long-term risks.

A good example would be going on a raw, freshly made fruit and vegetable juice cleanse. It will do its trick in the short term, but in the long term, it will be harmful as you will soon discover when you read about raw food diets in this section.

A nourishing diet is the healthiest diet for the long term. It is based on sound principles and needs to contain nutrient-dense foods that your body can absorb easily. Different foods still need to be personally tested to ensure compatibility with you as your condition change with time.

This diet constantly adapts to your changing needs, the seasons and your location, all while using the best possible ingredients and preparation methods.

SAD—The Standard American Diet

It is SAD. Many health advocates rightly claim that the Standard American Diet, which is what most Americans consume—toxic and fast foods—is the cause of our rampant chronic diseases.

We have allowed ourselves to become duped into believing that the cheapest, fastest food is okay to eat and that there are no consequences for living this lifestyle and eating C.R.A.P.—caffeine, refined sugars, alcohol and processed foods.

Then there is the meat that has massive amounts of hormones, anti-biotics and fear-based hormones released during factory slaughter; there are the toxic chemical fertilizers in our agricultural soils and on our fruits, vegetables and grains; there are men who have dangerously low sperm counts, infants who start life with inherited chemicals, and breast milk that is toxic and unsafe for our babies' consumption.

Our government agencies **do not** protect us. They have become a conduit for special interest groups that put the financial health of corporations ahead of human safety and real health.

As consumers, we have played along and have believed the commercials, the agencies and the businesses that tell us all is well with our food. We shirk our responsibilities to our own health by ignoring the evidence all around us.

We let our health degenerate to a level that is killing us and robbing our nation; government funds end up paying for treatment of chronic diseases that could have been avoided by making conscious and healthy choices. Even many of the so-called healthy choices advocated by mainstream nutritionists are a lie when you really examine what is in them.

Sadly, our Standard American Diet has become the *Sick American Diet*. It is the reason we have unprecedented rates of chronic disease. Sure you can take pills, be irradiated, or get surgery and call that a "cure" so you can continue the same old destructive patterns, but that is a joke.

A **real** cure must get to the root causes of the problem; otherwise, it is just a temporary treatment to cover up symptoms.

Prostate disease, along with all the other chronic health problems, is a disease of our ignorance. Sadly again, there is no bliss in this ignorance. An increasing loss of vibrancy replaces vitality and a pain-free, fully-functioning healthy life until an old age.

The great news is you can become educated and can put your SAD to an end—it is the only realistic solution. We make changes day by day, bit by bit. We STOP, CLEANSE and REVITALIZE by choosing the healthiest foods and products that we can.

Each of us needs to become aware of our choices and become our own caregiver. The Prostate Health Diet lays out suggestions for you to embrace these changes with the promise of a renewed and healthy you with a zap in your sex life and peeing that flows strong and long!

USDA Diet

Since the U.S. Department of Agriculture came out with their food pyramid in 1980, rates of obesity have skyrocketed.

Fats, Oils & Sweets — Use Sparingly

Milk, Yogurt & Cheese 2–3 Servings

Lean Meat, Poultry, Fish, Dry Beans, Eggs & Nuts 2–3 Servings

Vegetables 3–5 Servings

Fruits 2–4 Servings

Bread, Cereal, Rice & Pasta 6–11 Servings

Source: U.S. Department of Agriculture, 1992. Food Pyramid. www.peppercornpress.com

In 2011, the U.S. government replaced their food pyramid with MyPlate, as seen on the next page.

The USDA admitted in 2010 that the Food Pyramid diet was never tested and that it was developed to meet calorie needs rather than nutrient needs. Yet, many nutritionists were repeatedly finding that not only their patients, but they themselves, were becoming overweight, obese and sick while doing their best to follow the USDA's grain-based, carbohydrate-rich diets.

The major problems with this diet are:

- the use of excess refined carbs and sugars
- the lack of high quality nutrient rich oils and fats replaced by modern processed harmful vegetable fats
- the use of pasteurized and homogenized dairy
- poorly prepared whole grains and pulses and nuts

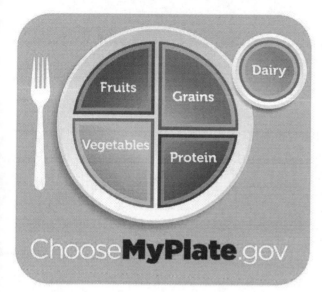

Source: U.S. Government, 2011.
MyPlate. tiny.cc/o26wzw

When people began consuming foods that this diet recommended **not to eat**, patients felt better, had more energy and lost weight. Their overall health improved! Read more about what caused obesity to skyrocket in this fascinating article: *The USDA's Pyramid Scheme* (tiny.cc/2c7wzw).

Raw Food Diet

This diet craze is all about eating foods in their natural state without cooking, but allows for processing at low temperatures to dehydrate some foods. Replacing junk foods with raw organic foods is a big step in the right direction, but not the ultimate destination.

The theory is that raw foods contain many more enzymes than cooked foods—cooking supposedly kills many of those enzymes—and are, therefore, best eaten raw for optimum health.

This may be true to a point, but what I believe is missed here is that the key is what the body is <u>able to absorb</u>. Cooking makes many foods much more absorbable. So the question becomes: Which has the most net gain, cooked or raw?

Most of the world's population today use cooked foods not raw, even in warm climates. (One exception is the practice of aboriginal peoples who eat raw meat after a kill in hunting: the liver, fat, heart and kidneys are the choice pieces for gaining power and nutrients.)

Why is it that virtually all primitive cultures cooked most of their food? The reason is to make the food more digestible by removing harmful anti-nutrients sometimes found in raw plant food and to optimize nutrient absorption.

In *Timeless Secrets of Health and Rejuvenation*, Andreas Moritz did a great job critiquing this raw food diet. He explained why it seems to work for a while, but described some of the very real risks in this way of eating long term. Raw foods can trigger a weakening of the digestive system after an initial cleansing of the colon, bloating, deterioration of joints and arteries, a weakened condition overall and the inability to absorb the very nutrients that raw foods possess. Moritz said, "To avoid the natural poisons contained in many raw foods, all major ancient civilizations traditionally prepared their foods." (amzn.to/n71lG7)

Scientists now conclude that the invention of using fire to cook food about a million years ago was what led to the growth of the human brain because cooked food allowed for greater nutrient absorption. This freed up nutrients to feed and nourish the brain leading to its major increase in size.

"Heating our food unlocked nutrition: 100 percent of a cooked meal is metabolized by the body, whereas raw foods yield just 30 or 40 percent of their nutrients." *What Makes Us Human? Cooking, Study Says* (tiny.cc/8g7wzw).

"Meat and cooked foods were needed to provide the necessary calorie boost to feed a growing brain." *Sorry, Vegans: Eating Meat and Cooking Food is How Humans Got Their Big Brains* (tiny.cc/vk7wzw)

Moritz went on to say, "The initial boost in energy and vitality after going on a raw food diet is not due to the vitamins; it is rather caused by the sudden mobilization of the immune system, which tries to counteract the massive influx of enzyme inhibitors and antibodies contained in the [raw] food."

Plant foods contain many anti-nutrients to protect them from predators. Traditional cultures knew that for their health, food had to be cooked, soaked or fermented. This is especially important for grains, nuts and beans.

That said, for some people coming off a toxic diet, the best choice may be a raw food **cleansing diet** for a while as it can help detox the body. However, a raw food diet may not be a healthy long-term choice, except for the strongest of constitutions. Perhaps mixed with some cooked food, it would be more balanced. Most raw foodists are also vegans, which has other risks added to the mix.

Raw foodists also eat sprouted foods. Sprouting does make foods more digestible but not as much as soaking the foods longer and cooking them. People who only eat raw foods also like eating "greens" in the form of sprouts like wheat grass or in dried powdered forms. Watch out—these types of green foods can be a real irritant. I have had complete prostate/urinary shutdowns by taking powdered greens, which were supposedly super healthy!

This diet seems to be best suited to certain geographic climates. Eating raw in more northerly climates in the winter will be a challenge as you could easily weaken your condition. Eating food "in season" is also something to take into consideration. Eating mangos regularly in Alaska in January may not be the perfect food! Personally test fruits that come from far away, and you may be surprised to get a NO.

Eating raw foods like sauerkraut or fermented veggies as part of a healthy, cooked food diet can accomplish what the raw food diet tries to do—maximizing enzymes. These foods are great sources of enzymes, which help digestion in the upper stomach where digestive fluids are lacking.

Lacto-fermentation (a fermentation process) improves the amount of enzymes in raw food and when eaten with cooked food compensates for the loss of enzymes in the cooked food, and can make it far easier to digest. This fermentation process also provides lactic acid and good bacteria that survive the digestion process and make it into the intestines. Lacto-fermented foods can be considered "super-raw."

Too many raw foods eaten when you are not absorbing vitamin D from the sun will be very hard on your body because raw foods, especially tropical fruits high in potassium, tell your body not to release extra vitamin D that your body needs to digest them.

The food itself—because of the high potassium content—signals that you are getting the vitamin D from the sun and that no more is needed, as we explained earlier.

This would work fine if you were in the tropics and out in the sun, not indoors. But it doesn't work in other climates if you are not getting D from the sun. As a result, your ileocecal valve (between your large and small intestines) eventually does not close fully and your whole digestive system is compromised as a result. So even the finest quality foods can become your enemy if not prepared properly!

My take on the raw food diet is to eat raw foods in moderation especially in winter in more northerly zones. Personally test (see Chapter 9) the raw food to know if it is good for you and how much to have. Raw foods may be useful for a while in order to cleanse, but once that initial stage is over, you may be creating a whole new set of health conditions. Return to cooking most of your foods. For me, I can eat apples raw from my own apple trees only in the late summer and early fall. After that I start to react to them. Once cooked into apple sauce, they are fine.

Most of us need to eat a lot more vegetables. Cooked is best for most of them, while salads and raw vegetable juices are fine in moderation.

Be very careful not to indulge in raw fruit juices except as a special occasion treat because of the high sugar content in fruit juices. Fruit is best eaten in its whole form so you get all the fiber and bulk nutrients.

The Vegetarian Diet

The vegetarian diet is a very popular diet with many variations and is claimed to be superior by many. However, many weaknesses have been found in this diet. For example, eating the wrong kind of dairy (i.e., pasteurized) will be harmful over time. Many vegetarians consume too many sweets and phytic rich grains, nuts and pulses poorly prepared. Vegetarians can become quite unhealthy. Life expectancy is significantly longer for wider-eating peoples of northern India (who also eat animal foods) than vegetarian peoples of southern India.

Vegetarians are often deficient in vitamin B12 because it is not found in plant-based foods. For more information, you can read *Vitamin B12: Vital Nutrient for Good Health* (tiny.cc/6p7wzw).

You can easily test non-vegetarian foods like eggs, fish, fowl and red meat to see if these foods test positive for you. If so, then you may well need them in your diet! If you need meat, eat high quality, grass-fed organic meat products.

To read more about the dangers of the vegetarian diet, read these articles:

Twenty-Two Reasons to Not Go Vegetarian (tiny.cc/0s9wzw)

Vegetarianism and Nutrient Deficiencies (tiny.cc/3u9wzw)

The Vegetarian Myth by Lierre Keith (tiny.cc/2v9wzw)

Lierre Keith described the dangers of a vegetarian diet not only to our health, but even more importantly, she destroyed the long-held myths of its supposed benefits to the environment and the ending of poverty.

She clearly showed that the current practices of mono-crop agriculture (never mind the prison-like factory farms for animals) have depleted well over 90% of the U.S.'s topsoil and threatens the survival of countless species.

Keith's book is an eye-opener and a must-read for anybody who cares about our planet and their own health. The book's subtitle should be: How our Agricultural Practices and Food Choices are Destroying the Planet and our Health!

Hey, I was mostly vegan/vegetarian for decades and I paid the price—I developed a prostate problem! So, if you are vegetarian, you may want to consider the near impossible: some animal foods of the right kind may be very beneficial for you and the planet!

Vegan Diet

This is essentially a vegetarian diet but without animal products, such as dairy or eggs, that vegetarians often eat. This diet often includes a large raw food component. Please see the above "Vegetarian Diet" for information on vitamin and nutrient deficiencies.

The China Study Diet

This is essentially a vegetarian diet, but without the animal products—such as dairy or eggs—that vegetarians often eat. This diet often includes a large raw food component. Please see the above diets (raw and vegetarian) for information on vitamin and nutrient deficiencies.

The China Study diet claims that rural Chinese are healthier because of their vegetarian/vegan diet. The reality is that many of the conclusions of this diet are based on false premises or science. For an excellent insight and analysis of its claims read *The China Study Myth* (tiny.cc/t09wzw).

Macrobiotic Diet

This diet is a variation of the vegan diet with some fish allowed and lots of grains, beans, nuts, seeds, vegetables and sea vegetables. Basically, it's a high complex carbohydrate, low fat, natural foods diet with no dairy.

I now know that many of these recommended natural, whole foods contain phytic acid. Also known as phytates, these anti-nutrients are so harmful over time if you don't remove them by traditional methods of soaking and fermenting. I only discovered this recently, and I believe that phytic acid has been the major factor in causing my enlarged prostate while I was eating a supposed healthy diet!

See the section on phytic acid in Chapter 2 and also Wikipedia's webpage for more info on *Phytic Acid* (tiny.cc/x29wzw).

Please note that the macrobiotic diet slowly removes zinc (and other minerals) from the body by not preparing foods properly. Zinc is a crucial mineral for the prostate. I had been mostly macrobiotic for well over 30 years, never knowing the dangers of that diet that I know now.

Alkaline Diet

Also known as the acid/alkaline or pH diet, this diet is growing in popularity. Food is categorized on whether it is alkaline or acid-forming in the body. I would rate this as a cleansing diet, **not** a long-term nourishing diet.

The goal of this diet is to eat foods so that the body maintains an alkaline state. The reason claimed is that an acidic state is the cause of many of our modern diseases and cancers. Most of the foods on my Food STOP List (see Chapter 5)—and in my lower levels of healthy eating—are too acidic.

An ideal alkaline diet, they say, is one that is largely vegetarian or vegan, and often raw, with at most small portions of animal foods. It also minimizes most grain and bean products because most are too acidic.

The goal is to eat approximately 75% of foods from the alkaline list and only 25% from the acidic list. Many claim successful healing of diseases and cancer with this diet.

You will find variations from different pundits on what constitutes the degree of acidity/alkalinity of a particular food, but experts seem to agree with each other's assessments on the bulk of the foods. Perhaps the best chart can be downloaded here: *List of Alkaline Foods* (tiny.cc/q49wzw).

Go here for more in-depth information:

Acid/Alkaline Diet (www.acidalkalinediet.net/)

The Alkaline Diet (www.thealkalinediet.org/course.html)

This diet may be beneficial for a short period as a cleansing diet, especially after a long-term diet of poor quality, manufactured foods but, in my opinion, this diet is harmful in the long term. The immediate benefits are felt, but in the long term, people on an alkaline diet may suffer as do many raw food vegans and vegetarians.

Eating an alkaline diet for a while will provide many more nutrients, but the restrictions on saturated fat may become costly over time as you are unable to absorb much of those nutrients. And if you do eat most foods in raw form then you will be harming your health over time (see the section on the raw food diet for explanation).

It's what we absorb and what minerals are maintained by the body that is the essential key to health, not the acid content of foods.

Another problem missed in this diet is simply that the wrong food for someone—even from the high alkaline group—can easily cause a negative reaction in the body, an acid-forming reaction because of the inflammatory response it causes. That's what happened to me when I ate kale, the highly recommended and very alkaline veggie. There are some people who just cannot tolerate that food.

Look at this conclusion from an amazing researcher, Dr. Weston Price, who studied the diets of primitive Swiss, Gaelic, Eskimo, Native American and South Sea Islanders. Dr. Price compared the amount of acid ash and alkaline ash minerals, and he wrote:

> *In all but the South Sea diet, acid ash foods predominated. But the important point is that the overall mineral content in every primitive diet was at least four times, and sometimes more than ten times, higher than the mineral content in the modernized diet.*
>
> *The Right Price by S. Fallon,* tiny.cc/fwnzzw

Note the date of that article—1935. Imagine how much more the modern diet would be depleted of minerals these days! My best advice is to use this alkaline diet as a transition cleansing diet and to personally test all the foods (read about *Personal Testing* in Chapter 9).

Low Glycemic Diet/South Beach Diet

This diet uses what proponents believe is the perfect guide: the glycemic index of foods. The Glycemic Index (GI) is a numerical scale used to indicate how fast and how high a particular food can raise your blood glucose (blood sugar) level. Supposedly, the lower the GI, the better that food is. You can read more here: *Glycemic Index on Wikipedia* (tiny.cc/8baxzw).

To me, the whole concept of GI is flawed because it classifies foods made with whole grains, such as rye bread, as being identical to jelly beans! Something is off base here!

Diets based on low glycemic index foods ignore two important facts: fats lower the glycemic index and so does cooking time! Put butter on your pre-soaked and cooked rice or on whole grain sourdough bread, and the glycemic index of these foods comes down, which means that these foods are absorbed slowly into the bloodstream rather than in one quick burst, which is what supposedly happens with high-GI foods.

Properly prepared foods with high quality saturated fats are what count, not some scientific diet! You can personally test to see whether your body wants some of the top quality, high-GI foods. Just prepare them properly and add good quality fats to help them be slowly absorbed.

Body Type Diets: Ayurvedic Diet/Blood Type Diet

The Ayurvedic diet is a time-tested and traditional diet based on Ayurvedic principles from India. It describes three basic body types and shows which foods are best for each body type and why. It has a lot of wisdom to teach us.

Here are three books about this diet. You can easily determine which body type you are from the questionnaires.

Timeless Secrets of Health and Rejuvenation (amzn.to/n71lG7)

Ayurvedic Healing, 2nd Revised and Enlarged Edition: A Comprehensive Guide (amzn.to/okRlD4)

Ageless Body, Timeless Mind: The Quantum Alternative to Growing Old (amzn.to/nkEzy0)

The Ayurvedic diet is largely vegetarian in its recommendations, so please do personally test the foods to confirm the suggestions; otherwise, with time, it could be too restrictive. I could not follow that diet today without reactions, especially since many phytate foods are recommended. Make sure you read the information on phytic acid reduction (see *Anti-Nutrients* in Chapter 2) to learn how to minimize this anti-nutrient.

Also, there are often too many tropical foods recommended in the Ayurvedic diet regime; we know that in raw form that can be a real problem in all but hot climates (see *Eat According to Your Climate* in Chapter 2).

It is a good starting point once you know your "type," but you still need to be careful with the recommendations. Take some ideas from the diet and then personally test the foods for your compatibility. Of course, no theoretical body type can account for the infinite varieties of body types that exist. In fact, Ayurveda expands the basic 3 to 10 versions.

The same cautions hold true for the blood type diet. This diet uses your blood type to tell you what to eat. Again, it's a scientific theory like the alkaline diet. But do make sure to take it with a grain of salt and test first!

Many of my blood body type food recommendations do not work for me as they test negative when I personally test or have immediate reactions if I eat them. The reality is your uniqueness. That is why diet theories just do not work over the long term.

Read more about the *Blood Type Diet* by Dr. Lam at this link: www.drlam.com/blood_type_diet/

Personally test foods for compatibility—you will know what resonates for you, and you will be amazed at what works for you. Your body's inner wisdom knows what it needs (see Chapter 9).

High-Carb-Low-Fat Diet or Low-Protein Diet; the Hunter-Gatherer Diet, Primitive Diet, or Paleo Diet; and the Low-Carb-High-Protein Diet

I am grouping these diets together because the questions of fat, protein and carbohydrates are common to all.

Weston Price, the researcher who was quoted above, has said that the high-carb-low-fat diet is risky. People who live in industrialized societies, as we do today, consume non-fermented carbohydrates and avoid nutrient-dense foods. They have a difficult time avoiding highly refined and devitalized food because these foods are everywhere. A diet comprised of these foods is completely out of balance and can be addictive because of additives designed to hook you!

Read CBC's article called *Food Cravings Engineered by Industry* (tiny.cc/cuaxzw), and this one by Natural News: *The Ultimate Craving—How Industry Designs Food to be as Addictive as Narcotics* (tiny.cc/rvaxzw).

Many now claim that the high-carb-low-fat diet is one of the main causes of the dramatic increase in obesity in the past 3 decades. The combination of too many devitalized carb starches in the white flour and sugar products we eat and the lack of proper fat to help digest them is deadly.

The Paleo diet says that we should eat what our ancestors ate before the advent of agriculture about 10,000 years ago. Enthusiasts claim that the Paleo diet was low in carbs and high in protein from meat and fish. The modern version often recommends lean cuts of meats. The result is, in fact, a diet very different from what our ancestors ate because it contains too little fat and too much protein, resulting in deficiencies.

The best Paleo diets suggest having adequate saturated fat and not to focus on lean meats, but these diet enthusiasts still have a problem with carbs.

Enthusiasts claim that carbs were not eaten back then but, in fact, roots and tubers were a mainstay of primitive diets, rich in digestible carbs when properly prepared and were eaten with saturated natural fats.

The problem is similar to the low-carb-high-protein diets:

> *Dieters often add protein powders to up the protein content without adding too many calories at the same time. The result can be a diet unnaturally high in protein, something that all primitive peoples avoided. Protein requires vitamin A for its metabolism and a diet too high in protein without adequate fat rapidly depletes vitamin A stores, leading to serious consequences—heart arrhythmias, kidney problems, autoimmune disease and thyroid disorders. Diets too high in protein also cause a negative calcium balance, where more calcium is lost compared to the amount taken in, a condition that can lead to bone loss and nervous system disorders.*
>
> *Adventures in Macro-Nutrient Land by S. Fallon and M. G. Enig* (tiny.cc/4obxzw)

The high protein weight loss diet will give good short-term results. You will lose weight. But in the longer term your body will become toxic (ketosis) from such excessive amounts of protein. You are asking for trouble such as kidney failure and kidney stones, cancer, organ failure, high cholesterol, osteoporosis and more!

The bottom line on these diets is that they are better than eating the way most Americans currently eat, which is mainly consuming foods that are on my Food STOP List (see Chapter 5). But are these diets ideal for you? The only way to know is to pay attention to their shortcomings and to personally test the foods (see Chapter 9).

As long as carbs in the form of whole grains and beans are prepared traditionally (soaked, sprouted, fermented, leavened) and are eaten with the best saturated fats, they become highly nutritious foods, assuming they test positive for you.

The other major problem with some of these diets is that they either recommend low-fat foods or vegetable fats instead of saturated fats. The vegetable fats have too high a ratio of omega-6 fats and, if these fats are from the Food STOP List, they can be very harmful. There will be more about the dangers of a low-fat diet later. For more insights on low fat diets, read this article: *Low Fat Diet Missing Essential Brain Nutrients and Leads to Cognitive Decline* (tiny.cc/hrbxzw).

The Weston A. Price Foundation's "Health Topics" is a most comprehensive site of research that investigates the best foods to eat. It is well worth the time to review and to search the site (tiny.cc/xtbxzw).

Again, I want to remind you that when you are researching online, no matter what great research and insights you find, the final test is to personally test foods before eating them.

Mediterranean Diets

These diets, eating the way cultures around the Mediterranean eat, may have some good points, but many incorrect conclusions have been drawn about fat and meat.

They recommend olive oil, an excellent occasional oil but not for constant primary use, and deny the benefits of high quality saturated fats. Many also want you to limit the intake of meats. A good idea for commercial varieties but leaving out traditionally raised animal products may harm you. The question of dairy also is crucial failing to understand the difference between pasteurized and raw milk dairy products.

See the discussion later in this book about these most important diet issues—fat, meat and dairy.

While excellent on the use of lots of vegetables, much of the grains used in these diets are highly refined with the nutrients removed; the pastas and breads are now white or are not prepared properly as we have discussed. See gluten-free diets below.

Weight Loss Diets

Be very careful with many of these programs that sell you protein shakes, powders and concoctions. Many of them are made with highly manufactured ingredients, which contain GMO derivatives of corn, soy and taste enhancers (neurotoxic ingredients). Many also use fructose sweeteners or artificial ones. Both of these sweeteners are highly toxic to your health.

> The FDA lists more than ninety documented symptoms of aspartame toxicity, including abdominal pain, anxiety attacks, brain cancer, breathing difficulties, chronic fatigue, depression, headaches, migraines, dizziness, marked personality changes, memory loss, panic attacks, rapid heartbeat, vision loss and weight gain. Sucralose side effects include rashes, panic attacks, dizziness, numbness, diarrhea, swelling, headaches, cramping and stomach pain.

> Dairy Industry Petitions FDA to Approve Aspartame by The Weston A. Price Foundation (tiny.cc/cvbxzw)

Another article is Aspartame Pathway (tiny.cc/xwbxzw).

Watch out for the so-called "diet" foods and protein energy bars. Most contain artificial sweeteners like Equal and Splenda. Both cause neurological damage, gastrointestinal problems and endocrine disruption.

Watch out for the added chemical flavoring agents. They take the place of fat and other natural components that have been removed to create an artificially reduced calorie level to fool you (www.naturalnews.com/natural.html).

Some people get great results using a cleansing diet (i.e., raw juice) and think that is the answer. But as we have already discussed, a cleansing diet isn't for the long-term because it becomes problematic at some point. Most dieters either get new symptoms or revert back to their old ways because they are not being nourished properly.

If you want to lose weight, follow the diet recommendations in this book. For permanent weight loss, a nourishing natural diet is the only way to sustain your optimum weight level.

Gluten-free Diets

Years of eating modern, processed grains that contain gluten—such as wheat, spelt, kamut, rye, oats and barley—can be very harmful to many people. The solution is to eat a diet that avoids gluten completely, say the proponents of this diet.

If you are sensitive to gluten, you will benefit from this practice in the short term. In the long term, there may be many risks in the gluten-free foods recommended. Unless gluten-free grains like rice are prepared by soaking to reduce the anti-nutrients (phytic acid), new conditions will develop.

Many of the gluten-free products being sold today in health food stores and supermarkets are loaded with poor quality ingredients: vegetable fats, sugars or substitutes, commercial eggs and GMOs. White rice is used frequently but is stripped of its nutrients, thus causing weight gain.

Many who are gluten intolerant probably developed this condition because of:

- the poor quality of modern commercial grains sold as white bread, pastas, etc.

  They are toxic for your body because they have been stripped of virtually all vitamins, minerals, fiber and other important nutrients. Because of this, the body does not know how to properly digest and assimilate these so-called foods, which can lead to health problems. Refined white flour has also been bleached with chlorine and brominated with bromide, two poisonous chemicals that have been linked to causing thyroid and organ damage.

  Bread, and Why Avoid Most of It by Dr. Lawrence Wilson,
  drlwilson.com/ARTICLES/BREAD.htm

- the anti-nutrients (phytates) in them (especially bad in flaked and extruded puffed cereals like rice cakes)
- the whole grains prepared without soaking and fermenting
- the use of bran (very high in phytates), which is very harmful to the gut if not part of the whole grain properly prepared for optimum digestion—avoid bran cereals!
- the lack of high quality saturated fats, such as butter from pastured cows, in the diet to help digest the grains and minimize any negative reactions

In fact, once you return to the proper preparation of whole grains with gluten, you may well find you can slowly start to introduce them into your diet!

That happened to me. After 35 years of eating grains without knowing how to safely prepare them and to add butter to help digest them, I had to cut them out of my diet completely. This lasted for a year. Gluten grains were the worst. But 2 years later, the only grains I can eat are wheat, rye and kamut as long as I prepare them properly! They contain a lot of gluten! I still cannot eat the gluten free grains like quinoa, and only limited amounts of carefully soaked brown rice very occasionally.

Conclusion

To conclude, many popular diets have some good ideas, but none will work for everyone. And many of them have serious flaws that will worsen your health. Take the advice of pundits with a grain of salt, glean what you can, then personally test every food to see if it works for your unique body (see Chapter 9).

In the next chapter's STOP lists, I review things that you most definitely should avoid.

Chapter 5: The "STOP" Lists

This section summarizes what to stop eating. Food is medicine and crucial to ensuring good health. We can choose not to become victims of our daily bad health habits.

Many of the bad foods we eat are addictive and toxic. Toxins are forced into our body's exterior tissues because not all of the toxins can be eliminated by the overburdened system of elimination. Weight gain is the result.

Our guts become a toxic wasteland and our digestion suffers. Chronic health conditions take root. Our prostates bear a huge burden. Eliminating toxic foods is essential to give your body a chance at natural healing. Review this list and see if it makes sense to you.

Sensitivities and Allergies

Chronic health conditions are the day-to-day ailments that afflict most people rather than a sudden disease or infection. Chronic ailments are closely related to sensitivities and allergies. It isn't any secret among practitioners in the natural health field that most patients who come to them with a long-term or chronic issue suffer from one or more allergies.

What exactly is an allergy? Allergies occur when the body's immune system produces antibodies, which is a response to the body's repeated exposure to a substance or antigen that is normally harmless.

The location in which the defense reaction is more noticeable in the body is where disruptive and uncomfortable symptoms will be most intense. For example, extreme mucus congestion and breathing difficulties arise if the reaction is in the nose, sinuses or lungs.

In the prostate, an allergic immune reaction could lead to an enlarged prostate. For women, a similar immune response may cause ovarian cysts.

If you have a toxic diet and suffer from constipation, you can imagine the time this sluggish elimination provides for toxic absorption across the thin rectal wall into the prostate. Every time you pee, toxins pass right through your prostate. What you eat counts big time!

The Gut

The more I have learned about healing, the more I realize how crucial our gut—our digestion—is for our health and the progress we make.

Most, if not all of us, have a very compromised digestive system. This sad state of affairs is caused by decades of abuse from inoculations, antibiotics, excess sugars, pesticides and chemicals, manufactured non-foods and anti-nutrients from foods not prepared properly.

If you have any of these symptoms then the culprit is most likely that your digestion is compromised, often known as 'leaky gut.'

- constipation or bloated stomach
- diarrhea or irregular bowels
- coated and/or sore tongue
- frequent gas or cramping
- awful-smelling bowel movements
- stomach aches and hemorrhoids
- bad breath or heartburn

If these symptoms occur frequently, it's a sure sign that your intestinal tract and colon are not functioning optimally.

Dangerous toxins build up in your bowels. This can easily trigger food sensitivities and allergies and more serious health conditions.

Antibiotics kill the bad and the good flora from your intestines, leaving your digestion in a very compromised condition. Your gut flora prevents overeating. Too much antibiotic use can strip the flora away, which can then result in chronic overeating!

Antibiotics take a terrible toll on the body's digestive system. Yes, at times they are essential and can save us from major health consequences. But in 90% of cases today, antibiotic use is out of hand and prescribed far too frequently for minor ailments. Every drug has a side effect.

Moral of the story: almost everyone has a compromised digestive tract. Whenever we use such strong meds on less than crucial purposes, we pay the price in terms of allergies, sensitivities, chronic health problems and a tired body that takes the pleasure out of life.

When you start to change and improve your diet, progress in healing is not a straight line upwards! In fact, it can often be a difficult journey because our digestion has been so compromised.

The solution is to do all you can to build up the friendly bacteria in the gut so that it can destroy some of the unfriendly critters. You do this by optimizing your diet, personally testing for sensitive foods, taking probiotics like digestive enzymes and acidophilus, glutamine and FOS and even doing colonic cleansing.

If you have a candida yeast syndrome, the culprit is usually sugars of all kinds with the worst being fructose.

The centre of our immune system is in our gut. You need all the friendly bacteria possible from fermented foods such as natural yogurt, sauerkraut, kefir, kimchi, miso and sourdough bread. These friendly bacteria and probiotics will aid your digestion and help you on your healing path. Please start with very small amounts (½ teaspoon) of these foods if they personally test positive for you (see Chapter 9). Then increase slowly.

Your tongue will tell you how you are doing. If it is not pink and uncoated then you know you have work to do!

The Food STOP List

My Food STOP List should be followed as much as possible because these foods have become toxic, de-nourished, altered and processed so much that they have become almost alien to our bodies.

Once you know how to personally test foods, you can test these non-foods to see for yourself if they are good or bad for you to eat. As a general guideline, I strongly suggest that for your prostate health, you stop these "Non-Food" products:

- Stop eating commercial manufactured food. This includes: cookies, candies, muffins, cakes, breads, crackers, frozen dinners, soft drinks—whether of the sugar kind or artificial sweeteners—sauces, oils, white flour products, white rice and pasta. Basically, avoid most of what you find in today's supermarkets.
- Stop eating most commercial, conventionally-grown, pesticide-contaminated fruits and vegetables.
- Stop using refined sweeteners such as sugar, dextrose, glucose, high fructose corn syrup (recently found to contain mercury in over 40% of products tested by the FDA); bottled fruit juices, "energy drinks", etc.
- Stop using all sugar substitutes and artificial sweeteners like Aspartame and Splenda brands, etc.
- Stop eating all hydrogenated or partially hydrogenated fats, trans fats and oils no matter how "healthy" the marketing departments make them appear. This includes canola oil (the first GMO food made from toxic rapeseed oil), corn oil, soy oil, margarine, safflower oil and cottonseed oil. Replace with butter, ghee, lard, extra virgin coconut, olive and avocado oils. Learn more here *Know Your Fats* (tiny.cc/stcxzw) and here *Canola Oil is Another Victory of Food Technology over Common Sense* (tiny.cc/lucxzw). Read this article on the *Dangers of Soybean Oil* (tiny.cc/7vcxzw).
- Stop consuming commercial pasteurized and homogenized milk and dairy products. Replace with raw milk ones (ideal) or organic versions (not as beneficial as raw). Learn more at *A Campaign for Real Milk* (tiny.cc/excxzw).
- Stop eating commercial factory eggs, fowl, meat and processed meats of all kinds. Replace with organic or grass-fed, free-range products (ideal).
- Stop using commercial salt. Use sea salt instead.
- Beware of health food store products that contain many of the above restrictions. Many health food store foods are unhealthy.
- Stop consuming Genetically Modified (GMO) or Genetically Engineered (GE) and irradiated foods. The American Academy of Environmental Medicine has issued a warning urging the public to avoid them in this article: *Genetically Modified Foods* (tiny.cc/85dxzw).
- Stop eating commercially farmed salmon and fish unless organic—these fish are fed toxic feeds and antibiotics.
- Stop eating fish that are very high in mercury such as king mackerel, swordfish, tilefish, grouper, marlin, orange roughy, walleye and tuna.
- Eat these fish instead: catfish, clams, flounder, haddock (Atlantic), herring, mackerel (North Atlantic, chub), mullet, oysters, perch (ocean), plaice, pollock, salmon, sardine, scallop, shrimp, sole (Pacific), squid (calamari), tilapia, trout

44

(freshwater) and whitefish. See this consumer guide for a complete list of the best and worst fish, *Consumer Guide to Mercury in Fish* found at tiny.cc/16dxzw

- Stop consuming canned foods. Not only are the can linings toxic (coated with BPA), but also the food is devitalized and nutrient poor.
- Stop drinking caffeinated commercial products and drinks.
- Stop taking powdered protein concoctions and mixes.
- Stop eating commercial cereals, grains, nuts and seeds and granolas. They contain phytic acid (phytates), which depletes the body of vital minerals. These foods, including organic grains, nuts and seeds, must be soaked first to reduce this irritant. The worst foods in this category are extruded ones like puffed cereals and flakes (often coated with oils and sugars), rice cakes, shredded and bran cereals.
- Stop consuming soy products like soymilk, tofu, frozen soy desserts, etc., as they contain very high levels of phytic acid. They also cause many problems, especially related to hormones. It is okay to eat miso, tamari and tempeh, which are made from fermented soybeans. Use only organic brands as most non-organic ones are not only sprayed with herbicides and pesticides but also contain GMO soy. See this article called *Soy Alert* for more info (tiny.cc/k8dxzw), and this article called *Truth about Unfermented Soy and Its Harmful Effects* (tiny.cc/98dxzw).
- Stop fluoridated water. It depletes iodine from the body causing hypothyroidism and immune deficiency as well as weight gain and heart disease. See this article *Fluoridation: The Scam of the Century* (tiny.cc/zaexzw) and this article *Fluoride Depletes Iodine in the Body, Causing Hypothyroidism and Immune Deficiency* (tiny.cc/acexzw).
- Stop drinking chlorinated city water. Chlorine is highly toxic and can mix easily with other trace contaminants in the water to make highly carcinogenic chemicals. Remove chlorine and other toxins from your water.
- Stop eating BBQ'd meats with flames that burn the fats causing carcinogens (polycyclic aromatic hydrocarbons). Slow cook your meat instead.
- Stop eating commercial foods containing monosodium glutamate (MSG) and other food enhancers like vegetable protein, hydrolyzed protein, hydrolyzed plant protein, plant protein extract, sodium caseinate, calcium caseinate, yeast extract, textured protein, autolyzed yeast and hydrolyzed oat flour.
- Stop eating at fast food outlets whose foods contain massive amounts of Food STOP List products.
- Stop using aluminum cookware and non-stick cookware. Use stainless steel, cast iron, stoneware or glass and ceramic pots and pans instead.
- Stop smoking and stop drinking most distilled alcohol. Drink red wine and small brewery organic beers in moderation instead.
- Stop as many pharmaceuticals as possible and choose natural medicines for very temporary use instead.
- Stop getting vaccines. For more info, read this article on the dangers of vaccines and the impact on your immune system, *Vaccine Epidemic: How Corporate Greed, Biased Science, and Coercive Government Threaten Our Human Rights, Our Health, and Our Children* (tiny.cc/tdexzw).
- Stop using disposable coffee cups and foam take-out containers. These contain formaldehyde preservatives as well as styrene (another chemical additive), which have both been added to the federal government's list of known or suspected carcinogens in the *12th Report on Carcinogens* (tiny.cc/9eexzw).

- Stop using your microwave. It kills your food.

The Food STOP List contains the modern killer foods and the primary cause of epidemic levels of chronic disease and prostate problems today. We are overfed, undernourished and highly toxic to cannibals!

The good news is that when you replace toxic foods with real, whole foods, you gain back your health and discover how delicious and yummy real foods are! If you start to grow some of your own food then you will be eating fresh food with mouth-watering flavors.

Stop Eating Microwaved Food

The Russians did a lot of research on microwaves. Microwave cooking destroys the B complex, C and E vitamins that are linked with the prevention of cancer and heart disease. Microwaving also destroys trace minerals in your food. Microwave-cooked food is nutritionally useless. Increased rates of cancer cell formation were found in the blood of people eating microwave-cooked meals as well as increased rates of stomach and intestinal cancers.

In Andreas Moritz's *Timeless Secrets of Health and Rejuvenation*, he wrote,

> *Reporting for the Forensic Research Document of AREC Research, William P. Kopp now states: "The effects of microwaved food byproducts are long-term, permanent within the human body. Minerals, vitamins, and nutrients of all microwaved food is reduced or altered so that the human body gets little or no benefit, or the human body absorbs altered compounds that cannot be broken down . . ."*

> *In a classical experiment 2,000 cats were given only food and water that were previously placed in the microwave oven, even for just one minute. The foods selected were the most nutritious and natural ones available. **Within six weeks, all cats mysteriously died.** While investigating the surprising result of the test, it was discovered that, although the cats looked well fed, the cells in their bodies virtually contained no trace of nutrient-components. The cats literally starved to death, despite all the nutritious foods. Microwaves turned their food into deadly poison.*

> *Timeless Secrets of Health and Rejuvenation by A. Moritz,* (amzn.to/n71lG7)

Yes, I know it's fast and convenient, but microwaved water also kills plants dead, fast! If you would like to read more about the dangers of microwaved food, this article describes the deadly effects of microwaved water: *Experiment—Microwaved Water Kills Plants* (tiny.cc/rgexzw).

To read more about the dangers of microwave ovens, read *Ninety Percent of Homes Contain This Health Risk* (tiny.cc/fjexzw).

To read more about how microwave-food causes cancer, *Why and How Microwave Cooking Causes Cancer* (tiny.cc/alexzw).

Now imagine what microwaved food is doing to you and your prostate!

Cosmetics and Personal Care Items STOP List

Your skin is your body's largest organ and easily absorbs what you put on it. Cosmetics and body care products often contain very toxic chemicals, which are absorbed through your skin.

Then your kidneys and liver have to deal with the chemicals. These toxic chemicals will affect your prostate over time.

Even cosmetics and body care products labeled "natural" are suspect because the word is not held to any standard or code. The word "natural" in marketing is overused and misleading.

The only real way to know if a product is safe is to search the *SIRI MSDS Index* (www.hazard.com/msds/) for specific ingredients and to avoid these specific chemicals:

- cocoamide DEA, diethanolamine, TEA, triethanolamine, MEA
- mercury
- parabens
- propylene glycol, propylene oxide, polyethylene glycol
- petrolatum and coal tar
- phthalates
- sodium lauryl sulfate, sodium laureth sulfate
- sodium fluoride

Make sure your toothpaste, soaps, shaving cream, shampoos and conditioners, deodorants, aftershaves and anything else you use on your body does not add to your toxic load. Read the ingredients; distrust products without ingredients.

The Environmental Working Group has an incredible database of body care products from shampoos to cosmetics and sunscreens, all ranked according to toxicity. Now you can easily find safe ones and analyze the ones you are using: *EWG's Skin Deep Cosmetics Database* (www.ewg.org/skindeep/).

Also see *EWG's Sunscreen Guide* (www.ewg.org/2013sunscreen/) and their *Not So Sexy* (tiny.cc/cafxzw) report on the hidden chemicals in perfume and cologne.

To avoid prostate problems, avoid using conventional body care products. Get smart! Know what you are using.

Yes, safe products will cost more in dollars, but they will keep you healthy. In the long run, that saves a lot of money and unnecessary suffering! Read this article that gives a great perspective on the issue: *Heal Yourself in 15 Days by Cleaning up Your Skin Exposure* (tiny.cc/zcfxzw).

To find excellent sources of body care products from small-scale producers, visit the *Organic Consumer Association* website at www.organicconsumers.org/ or *Organic Body Care Products* from Amazon (tiny.cc/rffxzw).

My best advice is to find organic body care products from a manufacturer that you can trust **and** whose product personally tests positive for you (see *Personal Testing* in Chapter

9). To be safe, every now and then retest your body care products to ensure that minor ingredients don't have a negative reaction over time.

One of my favorite brands, which goes a long way for the dollar, is the exceptionally high quality and pure line of soaps and shampoos made by Dr. Bronner (www.drbronner.com/). Try the almond scent. It's my favorite.

Household Products STOP List

The same story holds for the dangers of household products from laundry detergent to dish liquids, from floor cleaners to air cleaners. Conventional and "natural" versions are highly toxic. If you think the water washes it away, think again. The fumes get into the air you breathe and seep through your skin. The remnants stay in your clothes and also penetrate through your skin.

Stopping the toxic onslaught is the first step to regaining your health and preventing prostate problems from occurring or growing worse. Remember how close the prostate is to the bladder and rectum. Your prostate can easily absorb toxins from these organs because of its proximity.

You don't have to believe me—educate yourself. Read this brief article on the chemicals found in the different rooms and products in your home: *Toxic Household Chemicals* (tiny.cc/6nfxzw), and then personally test them to ensure they are okay (see Chapter 9).

Here are the toxic household products that should be stopped.

- Stop using commercial laundry products and fabric softeners and wearing them next to your skin. Replace with organic versions that have safe ingredients.
- Stop using deadly mothballs. These are so toxic that they are banned in Europe. Use natural alternatives instead such as citronella, sandalwood, cloves camphor/eugenin, lavender or aromatic cedar. See this article for more info: *Get Rid of Moth Balls and Other Harmful Insecticides and Use Natural Alternatives* (tiny.cc/2pfxzw).
- Stop commercial household chemicals and cleansers of all kinds. Here is a list of safe and inexpensive alternatives: *Household Cleaners and Natural Products* (tiny.cc/nrfxzw).
- Stop using plastic containers for food storage with the numbers 3, 6 and 7 in the recycling codes on the bottom. Code #7 plastics often contain BPA, which mimics estrogen and is very harmful to the prostate. Use glass containers instead.
- Stop using commercial air fresheners and perfumed candles. Replace with essential oil diffusers and beeswax candles.
- None of these synthetic chemical ingredients in household products have been approved as safe for humans by the FDA. Be wary of anything that contacts your body. Replace all body care products with organic versions that have safe ingredients. For a review of which preservative ingredients are safe, see the *Young Again* website (tiny.cc/9tfxzw).

You may think this list is extreme, but the reality is we have compromised our health so drastically that it is time to go back to safe, time-tested products. Give your body a break! Stop the "death by a thousand cuts"!

In issue #75 of Vista Magazine, an article on chemicals states:

> *There are 80,000 chemicals that are registered for industrial use by the US Environmental Protection Agency. There are medical tests for only 250 of them. The health agencies have tested samples of people to try to assess the degree of contaminants in the average citizen. They tested for the presence of 210 chemicals and found 167 of them in the people tested. The average number of chemicals in any one person was 91.*
>
> *The obvious conclusion is that we are all toxic to one degree or another. It is no surprise that we are fighting a losing war on cancer, Alzheimer's disease, diabetes, thyroid disease, super bacterial infections and many other chronic degenerative conditions.*
>
> *The Obesity-Toxicity Connection* by S. Kuprowsky (tiny.cc/tvfxzw)

Go through your whole house and start to throw out the toxic household products. Replace all of these products with organic and healthful products. That's a lot of things to change and stop doing if you want to regain your health, but it is well worth the effort!

My favorite organic all-purpose super-concentrated household cleanser that you dilute in a spray bottle is called Orange TKO.

> *Orange TKO is a citrus cleaner/degreaser made from the peel of the orange. It is an emulsifier which contains no synthetic chemicals, petroleum distillates, or detergents. It is also 100% environmentally friendly, biodegradable, and non-toxic. Orange TKO comes as a concentrate which can be diluted with water to handle the toughest industrial cleaning problems, but is safe enough to use in the home, around children and animals. In the home, Orange TKO can be used for all of your cleaning applications.*
>
> *Dedicated to the Preservation of the Environment* by Orange TKO (www.tkoorange.com/)

Two quick tips on how to use this amazing cleaner: always shake the spray bottle before use. And let it sit for 10–30 seconds before wiping. TKO will then work like a charm, and it is inexpensive! Now you can throw out all your commercial toxic stuff.

If you want more information on the dangers of many common household materials, then take a look at this article: Common Household Materials Contains a Toxic Brew of Dangerous Chemicals.

Yikes! No wonder prostate disease is epidemic in the West!

Pest Problems?

Here is another safe household item to replace your toxic ones: AlwaysEco Pest Control Products. These products use completely organic, safe ingredients and at the same time are better than conventional toxic chemicals for your lawn and garden. They are also excellent for ridding your home of pests like wasps or bed bugs.

Purge your home! Get rid of all that nasty stuff. Fill your home with organic household products: Organic Household Products.

Do not overlook the role of household products on your health. If you want a healthy prostate, then there are no shortcuts. Use only safe products in your home.

Using Safe Cookware

Do you want to know more about which cookware is best to use?

> There's good reason why glass and ceramic beakers are used in a chemistry lab where it's critical that containers don't taint the experiment. Glass and ceramic are inert or non-reactive . . .

> My purpose is not to scare you but rather to help you realize why disease can develop based on our inputs. Knowledge is power. You start by making changes where you can, by substituting healthier choices little by little. Over time they will add up and your health will improve.

> Before making your next kitchen purchase, consider the reactivity of various tools and cookware and, whenever possible, favor inert or non-reactive.

Healthy Cookware by R. Wood, tiny.cc/w3nzzw

This article provides further evidence of the dangers of non-stick cookware: *Be Informed: Non-Stick Pans Pose Danger* (tiny.cc/brnzzw)

Here is a list of safe cookware with links to sources:

- Natural Stoneware Bakeware (tiny.cc/eqtky)
- Ceramic Cookware (tiny.cc/yzlod)
- Glass Cookware (tiny.cc/ynahi)
- Cast Iron Cookware (tiny.cc/rjaha)
- Stainless Steel Cookware (tiny.cc/8dm7f)

Conclusion

Yes—it is a challenge to change your old habits. All I can do is encourage you. The road ahead is clear if you want great health. The road you have been on leads to a destination you may no longer want. You decide the most important trip of your lifetime!

What I will suggest is that you revert to the foods of a hundred years ago before they were adulterated by insane food processing and agricultural practices that have created a toxic time bomb. In Chapter 6, I go into much greater detail about those healthy foods.

Chapter 6: The Whole Wide World of Food and What You Should Eat

Talk about a challenge to simplify all the conflicting information from a multitude of health sources and well-meaning practitioners. And, with our likes and dislikes, food is so personal for each of us. The task of figuring out what you should eat is a mighty one!

My approach is different from others in that the first rule is to eliminate all the well-known harmful foods first and then analyze the data on what foods are "best" for our health. Next, test what is best for you. **Knowing** is the final key that will set you on your road to health.

Let's see if we can agree on some principles.

- Food is powerful medicine, which can both heal and harm. Because food is our daily input that renews our cells, the quality of the food we consume has a direct impact on our health.
- Our food will help or harm us. Harmful effects can take time to be noticed or no time at all. Some people can eat horrible nutrient-poor, toxic food and not appear to suffer any consequences for years or decades, while others are so sensitive they can react right away to improper food. When the effects finally do surface—sometimes decades later—the severity of disease can be extreme.
- We are all so unique and different that every diet must be customized for each one of us. What is beneficial to me may be harmful for you. It doesn't matter how wonderful the research or popularity is on a particular food, herb or supplement. We are the master and must learn for ourselves what works, starting with broad guidelines and personal testing to verify them as helpful or harmful.
- Everything changes including our bodies, which change and require different inputs day by day. A food that is not good for you today may in fact be ideal on another day or year.
- What we consume is more than food; it also includes other inputs to our bodies such as liquids like water, substances that pass through our skin and the air we breathe.

Real Food List

When people eat real food on a daily basis, they are healthy and long-lived. This is evidenced by the isolated peoples found today in more remote places and mountains who practice the following time-proven habits:

- Eat meat from grass-fed, free-roaming, pastured animals and eat fowl that are free roaming and feed on scraps and insects.
- Eat eggs from birds that are free range and feed on scraps and insects; these eggs will be rich and healthy with deep yellow yokes.
- Eat vegetables and fruits grown in healthy soils, with no sprays and toxins added.
- Eat healthy fats and oils.
- Eat grains, beans, pulses and nuts and seeds prepared in the traditional manner of soaking, souring, or fermenting before cooking.

51

- Eat wild foods when they are in season (e.g., berries, mushrooms, nettles, etc.).
- Use real sea salt and eat some sea vegetables filled with trace elements and minerals.
- Use natural, minimally processed sweeteners from plants, bees and trees.
- Use spices and herbs and drink teas grown in home gardens or harvested locally.
- Drink clear, uncontaminated water.
- Breathe fresh unpolluted air filled with oxygen.
- Increase your exposure to natural sunlight.

Your prostate is your barometer of how healthy you are. Pay attention to its message and learn how to feed yourself for health and wellbeing.

The *Honest Food Guide* is not bad except for the fact that it doesn't discuss the differences between healthy grass-fed dairy, fats and meat. Ignore the soy recommendations: www.honestfoodguide.org/

Food is your medicine. A supplement cannot make up for the complex structures of nutrients that real food provides. **Real food** is the foundation of your health.

Fats

Fats are probably the most important food because of their potential to harm or heal us and because fats have the highest calorie content of all food groups; yet fats are a complex topic because there are so many viewpoints.

Today even mainstream medical organizations—not just holistic health sites—mistakenly say that to improve prostate health, people should reduce their fat consumption, especially the "deadly" saturated fats. Some assume that all fats are harmful and that all fats should be reduced.

It's true that today's mainstream saturated fats are toxic: various toxins, hormones and antibiotics concentrate even more in the fatty tissues of commercial, factory-farmed animals and in dairy fats. The more we consume these toxic foods, the more our disease rates and prostate problems explode. In fact, the highest rates of prostate disease occur in those countries that eat the most animal fat and animal foods.

Could it be that the **type** of fats and the toxins that reside in them are more harmful rather than the **amount** of fat we consume? To me, this is the essential question.

We need our fat to come from healthy, free-ranging, grass-fed animals and fowl not from animals that are poisoned by toxic chemical supplements in the feed, toxic antibiotics, pesticides, etc.

In traditional cultures, fat (mostly saturated fats) was revered for its health benefits as were the internal organs of an animal. Animal fat, butter and coconut oil are examples of saturated fat. Hunters survived poorly on a diet of rabbit that has very little fat, if they were the only animal they could kill in the winter.

For information on the dangers of low-fat diets, read this article: *Low Fat Diet Missing Essential Brain Nutrients and Leads to Cognitive Decline* (tiny.cc/eonzzw).

Take a look at this major study: In October 2010, the *American Journal of Clinical Nutrition* reported that saturated fats are NOT associated with an increased risk of coronary heart disease (CHD) including stroke or cardiovascular disease (CVD)!

> **Conclusions:** *A meta-analysis of prospective epidemiologic studies showed that there is no significant evidence for concluding that dietary saturated fat is associated with an increased risk of CHD [coronary heart disease] or CVD [cardiovascular disease].*
>
> *Meta-analysis of Prospective Cohort Studies Evaluating the Association of Saturated Fat with Cardiovascular Disease by P. W. Siri-Tarino, Q. Sun, F. B. Hu, and R. M. Krauss,* tiny.cc/rpnzzw

This conclusion destroys the myths of the supposed dangers of saturated fats. Taking this study's conclusions one step further, I believe that the rise of heart disease (and many chronic conditions like prostate disease) in modern societies should be attributed to:

1. the harmful, highly refined vegetable oils manufactured today and encouraged by virtually all government bodies and organizations like the American Cancer Society and the American Heart Association, which are against saturated fats; and

2. the changed nature of commercial saturated fats from modern agribiz methods with all its toxins and omega fat imbalances.

Good Fats to Eat

After years of following the advice of natural health pundits and experts, reducing my fat intake and eliminating saturated fat (eating a low-fat diet), my prostate still suffered and actually worsened the more diligently I stuck to the recommended path! I was following advice given by eminent practitioners with very successful practices who had well-researched and published information.

My conclusion is that these practitioners' recommendations are wrong because they only look at the surface of statistics; for example, "greater fat = greater prostate disease," which seems true on the surface, but it is wrongly concluded from the research. Like urologists who say that aging causes prostate disease, these practitioners are drawing the wrong conclusions from the data.

Remember: the problem is **not** the high quality, grass-fed fats, but the saturated fats from toxic animals and the modern vegetable fats that contain excessive omega-6s and toxins. Toxins and omega imbalances are the problem!

Eat nutrient-rich saturated fats like butter from free-grazing cows and coconut oil. Eat the natural meat fats with your good quality meat rather than lean cuts. Yes, this goes against all the propaganda!

Add to that healthy cod liver oil fats and rich fats found in wild salmon—these are the foods that nourished our ancestors throughout the ages.

Worried about cholesterol? Then read this book that dispels many of its myths being propagated today—*Ignore the Awkward: How the Cholesterol Myths Are Kept Alive* (tiny.cc/2g3yzw).

Read this article that exposes the myths that cholesterol from saturated fat is the major harbinger of heart disease and death: *You Have Been Lied to about Cholesterol and Fats* (tiny.cc/jj3yzw).

The use of quality saturated fat will be the most important decision you can make regarding fat. You can easily personally test to see if what I am saying is right for you (see Chapter 9). I bet you will find your body responds to high quality saturated fats with a big YES!

Then test the commercial fats (soy, corn, safflower and the margarines) and what you see will surprise you.

A wonderful source of the highest quality saturated fat from grass-fed cows is called ghee, or clarified butter. It is delicious and stable without refrigeration with a long shelf life. It is shipped unrefrigerated and packed in jars. Ghee is a great source of the best kind of saturated fat and is lactose free. You can use it plain or for cooking as it has a high smoke point. See the Pure Indian Foods website for more info (www.pureindianfoods.com/).

Omegas

Another thing to consider is the omega-6 to omega-3 ratio. It is the omega-3s that we are deficient in. The modern omega-6 to omega-3 fat ratio has become too extreme, and we are eating way too many omega-6s.

This reveals itself in aspects of our diet that we don't even think about such as meats purchased in your regular supermarket or restaurant. For example, grass-fed beef contains omega-6 and omega-3 fatty acids in close to the healthy 2:1 ratio. But grain-fattened commercial beef, which most people eat, contains fat in an imbalanced ratio—20:1, 30:1 and even 50:1 in favor of omega-6!

Omega-6 polyunsaturated fatty acids have a tumor-promoting effect whereas omega-3s have a protective effect.

See Jon Barron's article, *Fats and Oils Made Simple* (tiny.cc/xt3yzw).

Avoid These Bad Fats

Avoid the modern vegetable fats except olive, coconut and avocado oils and **always use extra virgin pressings of these oils**. Organic expeller-expressed sesame, peanut and flax oils are also okay, especially in salads, but I recommend using these oils in smaller quantities or for occasional use. Avoid commercial refined varieties of oils. Clearly, trans fats are highly processed and dangerous fats to consume.

Stop the soy, corn, safflower, sunflower, canola, hydrogenated and partially-hydrogenated oils and margarines completely, even the health food store or organic varieties. Ignore the mainstream marketing of how healthy they are for you! Here is another excellent article on fat: *The Great Con-ola* (tiny.cc/mv3yzw).

Margarine

Let's take a look at what goes into making margarine. Vegetable oils are heated to extremely high temperatures. This causes the oils to become rancid. A nickel catalyst is then added to the heated oils to ensure that the oils solidify. Deodorants and colorants are also added in this process.

> *The final solidification process creates harmful trans-fatty acids, which are highly carcinogenic. Margarine contains other extremely harmful ingredients such as emulsifiers, preservatives, free radicals, artificial flavors, bleach, soy protein isolate (MSG), sterols, and hexane, as well as many other artificial and synthetic ingredients. Hexane in itself should never be consumed, as it is derived from crude oil. Sterols are estrogen compounds which can cause endocrine problems and also have the ability to contribute to sexual inversion in animals. BHT (Butylated Hydroxytoluene) is used as a preservative in most margarine products. What is really concerning about this ingredient is that it is also linked to symptoms and side effects such as abdominal pain, dizziness, nausea and vomiting.*

> *Why Organic, Raw Butter will Benefit Your Health* by S. Botes, tiny.cc/yw3yzw

Eat More Fats!

Increase the amount of good fats in your diet! Yes, I said *increase* them! These were the revered foods of our ancestors. They prized the fat and internal organs of the animal for their rich nutrients. After a hunt, the internal organs were often eaten right away and raw for their richness. The lean cuts were fed to the dogs and only eaten when they had nothing else. Our ancestors knew what to eat to survive and thrive.

Dental and skeletal records show that pre-agricultural humans were taller and stronger, and they had no cavities compared to those after agriculture began. The amount of good fat was reduced in the diet of many as the population increased through agriculture and had limited access to the quality sources of nutrition.

Once our ancestors learned to ferment and soak grains, they were able to avoid the ravages of the phytic acid in those foods. But too much reliance on grains with a lack of the good fats led to a decline in health, which can also be seen in the skeletons and dental records.

Please read more here in this fascinating book: *An Edible History of Humanity* by Tom Standage (tiny.cc/xy3yzw).

> *Hunter-gatherers actually seem to have been much healthier than the earliest farmers . . . Farming results in a less varied and less balanced diet than hunting and gathering does . . . Cereal grains provide reliable calories, but they do not contain the full range of essential nutrients . . .*

> *Evidence from studies of bones reveals that farmers suffered from various diseases of malnutrition that were rare or absent in hunter-gatherers. These include rickets (vitamin D deficiency), scurvy (vitamin C deficiency), and anemia (iron deficiency). Farmers were also more susceptible to infectious diseases such as leprosy,*

tuberculosis, and malaria as a result of their settled lifestyles . . . As the farming groups settle down and grow larger, the incidence of malnutrition, parasitic diseases, and infectious diseases increases.

Not eating quality saturated fats with a high carb diet becomes deadly over time, increasing health problems as seen in these bone records and described earlier in our discussion on phytates.

We have also been led down a false path in the interests of false assumptions and corporate profitability promoting unhealthy highly processed oils (modern oils are extremely profitable to industry).

Since modern oils replaced our healthy fats and healthy animals were replaced with toxic, factory-farmed versions, we have begun to pay a huge price in our declining prostate health and increased cardiovascular disease. The Weston A. Price Foundation says:

> *Saturated fats are required for the nervous system to function properly, and over half the fat in the brain is saturated. Saturated fats also help suppress inflammation. Finally, saturated animal fats carry the vital fat-soluble vitamins A, D and K2, which we need in large amounts to be healthy.*
>
> *Human beings have been consuming saturated fats from animal products, milk products, and the tropical oils for thousands of years; it is the advent of modern processed vegetable oil that is associated with the epidemic of modern degenerative disease, not the consumption of saturated fats."*
>
> *Principles of Healthy Diets by The Weston A. Price Foundation*, tiny.cc/9z3yzw

Saturated fat—with a healthy omega 6:3 ratio—suppresses inflammation. This is a key benefit for reducing benign prostatic hyperplasia (BPH), the enlargement of the prostate, which is now epidemic in the modern world.

Summary on Good Fats

Saturated Fats

- Animal fats (from pastured animals) in meat and in butter, ghee and tropical oils (e.g., coconut oil and palm oil) contain primarily saturated fats.
- Daily saturated fat recommendation: 2–4 tablespoons.

Monounsaturated Fats

- Olive oil, sesame oil, peanut oil, avocado oil and nuts (e.g., almonds, cashews, walnuts, pecans, etc.) contain primarily monounsaturated fats.
- Daily monounsaturated fat recommendation: 1–2 tablespoons (or a small handful of nuts).

Polyunsaturated Fats

- Cod liver oil, flax oil, fish oils, evening primrose oil, black currant oil and borage oil contain primarily polyunsaturated fats.
- Daily polyunsaturated fat recommendation: 1–2 teaspoons.

Read this article called *The Skinny on Fats* if you want more info (tiny.cc/s33yzw). Remember to always choose organic extra virgin versions of the oils you eat.

Oil and Fat Smoke Points

When you cook with oil, you want to make sure that you do not allow the oil to reach its smoke point. When oil starts smoking, the oil transforms and can become a carcinogen (i.e., cancer causing). That is also why BBQ'd meats that flare because the oil catches fire are hazardous to you.

Below are oil smoke points of recommended oils sorted by temperature. Oils listed in **bold** font are suggested safe oils to use daily, use other oils on occasion, and omit oils not listed below because they are unsafe to use at any temperature (e.g., canola oil).

Temperature	Oil
225°F	Flaxseed Oil, Unrefined – *do not heat this oil!*
320°F	Peanut Oil, Unrefined; Walnut Oil, Unrefined
350°F	**Butter**; **Coconut Oil**; Sesame Oil, Unrefined
361–390°F	Lard; Olive Oil; Extra Virgin Macadamia Nut Oil
410°F	Sesame Oil
430°F	Almond Oil; Hazelnut Oil
440°F	Peanut Oil
482°F	Ghee
491°F	Avocado Oil, Unrefined

Protein

Protein is another controversial topic. We have so much invested in the notion that high protein is what we crave and need to be healthy. As discussed earlier, it is the quality fat we really need but have been told by the punditry to avoid. Worse yet, we are told to use commercial toxic fats and oils instead!

With adequate natural saturated fats, your cravings for protein will be reduced substantially. It is nutrient-rich broths with the animal fats, coconut oils and butter that will make a big difference to your metabolism.

The best solution is to test for the amount of protein your body needs through personal testing. Remember the portion size rule (in the section called *Meat*) or—better yet—personally test to determine the optimal amount of protein for you (see *Personal Testing*, Chapter 9).

If you are vegetarian, then ensure that any protein from dairy comes from grass-fed animals. Whole grains and beans, by the way, are excellent sources of high quality protein. Prepare your grains, beans, pulses, nuts and seeds by soaking or fermenting prior to sprouting or cooking to remove the harmful phytates. For more information about protein, read *Grass-fed Basics* (tiny.cc/k53yzw). Then find sources of grass-fed meat and dairy at this site: www.eatwild.com/index.html.

Poultry and Eggs

Choose organic, free-range products, as the commercial products are highly toxic from poor feed, confinement and manufacturing additives that are especially harmful to your prostate.

Commercial eggs have much more omega-6 fats than organic, free-range ones, which are higher in the beneficial omega-3 fats.

Some health gurus say that eggs are one of the worst foods you can eat and others the complete opposite such as this opinion article: *Eggs—Consume This Natural Protein Source* (tiny.cc/773yzw).

I recommend that you personally test to see if eggs are okay for you and how many eggs you can eat on a particular day.

Carbohydrates: Grains, Beans and Legumes

There are some health guru pundits of low-carb diets who claim that we need to avoid carbohydrates like grains, beans and legumes at all costs.

Some claim that primitive man did not eat carbs, but recent evidence shows that tubers, which are a carb, were eaten regularly in ancient times.

Today, so many of our carbs come from denatured, highly-processed grains in the form of white flours (e.g., breads, cakes, muffins, cookies, etc.) and from grains extruded with high-temperature processing (e.g., rice cakes, packaged cereals, etc.). These are deadly for the body. All the vitamins and minerals have been removed, and you are left with a nutritionless starch that is full of chemicals from agribiz farming.

What about other carbs, like whole grains and flours? While filled with nutrients, the problem with whole grains today—even organic grains—is the phytic acid in them, as we have said earlier. Also known as phytates, these anti-nutrients are difficult to digest and deplete your body of valuable minerals like calcium, iron, magnesium and zinc. (See Chapter 2 for more information.)

It is essential to remove the phytic acid in carbohydrates, which is easy to do. Soak your rice overnight or start soaking it in the morning for that evening's dinner, rinse, add fresh water and some sea salt and cook. They will cook in about half the time as unsoaked grains. If carbs are not a major portion of your diet and you eat them only occasionally, you may not feel the results of improper preparation. But it is still best to soak foods containing phytic acid.

The no- or low-carb diets are too extreme. The key is to prepare carbohydrates properly and to use the whole grain, not the devitalized processed ones. Avoiding this simple step defeats the many benefits of the goodness found in whole grains, beans and nuts and seeds.

Whole carbohydrates properly prepared provide rich minerals and nutrients, and they are very pleasurable to eat! Just add good saturated fat like organic butter to make them even more digestible and tasty.

Avoid all extruded grain products, even from whole grains, such as rice cakes and flaked and puffed cereals because they contain maximum phytates due to the high-temperature processing.

Many people are allergic to gluten in grains. If you are one of those, try soaking your grain or flour to see if you do better with phytate-reduced breads. The culprit could be that or the combination of the two: gluten and phytates.

You can personally test phytate-reduced breads to see if you can then tolerate the gluten. By making your own bread with fresh-ground flour properly soaked, you may be able to digest previously intolerable grain products. You can also try some of the ancient grains in the list below that are not gluten-rich such as kamut.

You can find some good information on whole grains on the *Whole Grains Council* website (tiny.cc/993yzw).

- amaranth
- barley
- buckwheat
- corn, including whole cornmeal and popcorn
- millet
- oats, including oatmeal
- quinoa
- rice, both brown rice and colored rice
- rye
- sorghum (also called milo)
- teff
- triticale
- wheat, including varieties such as spelt, emmer, farro, einkorn, kamut, durum and forms such as bulgur, cracked wheat and wheat berries
- wild rice

NOTE: When using any recipes make sure you first follow the phytic acid reducing soaking procedures first.

For a wonderful breakfast cereal try Ezekiel Cereals, instead of the high-heat extruded flakes and puffs that enhance the anti-nutrient phytic acid. Ezekiel Cereals are not high-heat extruded. This company sprouts the grains to reduce the phytates and then cooks them slowly at a low temperature to preserve good nutrients. They are packed with an amazing crunchy crunch to boot (tiny.cc/nb4yzw).

When cooking your beans or legumes after soaking, you can add a strip of kombu seaweed to further help reduce phytates in the cooking process. As an added benefit, both the soaking and the kombu reduce flatulence (farting).

Soy

Soybeans are high in phytates and must be well soaked and fermented to increase digestibility and nutrient absorption. Soy is a controversial food. Some proclaim it has many benefits and others warn of its dangers.

If you follow the food preparation guidelines from above, you can enjoy soy without any risks. Personal testing of these products is easy so you can be sure they are healthy for you to consume. I have also written more on this and have supplied articles in my Food Stop List

The Cornucopia Institute — Organic Soy Scorecard provides a list of the best producers of high quality soy products. I would only eat the products ranked with 4 or 5 stars and only those products that have been soaked or fermented (www.cornucopia.org/soysurvey/).

Read the articles *Is Soy Healthy* for more information about the risks of soy (tiny.cc/cb5yzw) and also this article, *Soy Dangers Summarized* (tiny.cc/ui5yzw).

You can get a complete breakdown of the many benefits of high quality carbs (i.e., grains, beans and legumes) here: *The World's Healthiest Foods* (whfoods.org/foodstoc.php).

Bread

One last note on phytates—if you love fresh bread, nothing beats grinding the flour from the whole grain. It is freshest this way and does not become rancid or lose vitamins as flours can easily do from sitting too long. In fact, it is best to refrigerate whole wheat flours. The other benefit of fresh grinding is the taste. So much better!

Here is how I use wheat. My pancake and sourdough recipe:

I hand grind my hard, spring, organic wheat berries into fresh flour thus retaining maximum nutrition (flours lose lots when pre-ground). Sometimes I add kamut and 10–15% rye berries, which are great at reducing the phytates in the other grains. Kamut and rye berries contain a lot of phytase so that when they are soaked, they do the phytate-reduction trick.

I then add water and mix in some whey (a tablespoon per cup of ground flour) from yogurt or some lemon juice. I let this sit on the counter overnight. In the morning, I pour off the top water in which a lot of the phytates now reside.

For pancakes, I add some ghee or butter or olive oil, an egg per cup or so of flour and ¼–½ teaspoon of baking soda, some sea salt and mix. You want quite a runny batch at this stage so that the pancakes are quite thin. Fry in a well-oiled, cast iron pan with some ghee ideally (perfect for frying because of higher smoke point).

Usually I make enough ground flour to have lots of soaked flour; I put aside about half of it to make sourdough bread. If you have a sourdough starter, then add it now and let it sit for another half to a whole day to ferment and bubble up. Then pour off the water from the surface the next morning.

Once a yeasty aroma develops, I then grind more fresh flour and add it to the mix with some sea salt. I form that into ball of dough, knead it for 5 minutes, then place it in a bowl covered with a damp cheesecloth. I often cut off some of the dough and roll it into chapattis, which are fried in a pan with some ghee for a yummy breakfast or lunch with added veggies and raw cheese. The rest of the dough sits until it rises nicely in the bowl for another half day or more. Then I knead that for 5–10 minutes and put in a baking bread pan to rise again. Once risen, I then have sourdough bread ready to bake at 350° for 35–40 minutes until it has a hollow sound when tapped on top.

Nothing compares to the taste and nutrient value of bread made this way! Add lots of butter when you eat it! I usually prefer to toast it for the best flavor. Preparing wheat this way may quite possibly be fine for gluten sensitive people. Test to know.

Meat

Let's take a closer look at meat. Meat today is so far removed from our natural meats of yesteryear that they have become killer foods with dangerous excesses of omega-6 fats.

For example, feeding grains to livestock rather than grazing the livestock increased the weight and milk production of animals. It also created a highly profitable industry.

In turn, consumers have been delivered meat and dairy products filled with hormones, antibiotics and imbalanced omega-6 to omega-3 ratios. Our daily consumption of these foods creates the conditions for our diseases: heart disease, cancers, diabetes and chronic health conditions such as allergies.

We eat poison! We have let our governments and industries deliver to us the lowest grade cheapest food possible without real concern for health.

All of that unhealthy food is certified as Grade A ("A" should be for "awful")! What has been done to our food supply is a travesty. Hey, your nose never lies. Have you ever driven by a factory cow or pig farm? The stench is unbearable! Think that food is healthy? Yum—bring it on!

Changes in hormonal balance are perhaps the key to the drastic rise in Western prostate conditions, including prostate cancer. So what causes this hormonal change? Doctors say it is a natural consequence of aging. Alternative practitioners often blame high fat, high dairy and high meat diets as the culprits.

I contend that it is none of the above! Rather it is the changed nature of the meat: grass-fed with added chemicals, antibiotics and growth hormones that alter once-healthy animal meat into toxic food for humans.

Meat can be an emotional issue for many people, especially vegans and vegetarians. I know because I was one for decades!

If you personally test YES for high quality, grass-fed, organic meat, avoid big slabs and eat it with some fat so you can ensure it is healthy for you. Here are some other guidelines:

1. Eat only meat from grass-fed, free-roaming, pastured animals—animals like they were meant to be. By law, New Zealand lamb must only be pasture raised. It is quite widely available.

   Avoid commercial toxic meat completely—it is deadly because of the feeds used and toxins, antibiotics and estrogens accumulated in the meat.

   Grain-fed organic beef, while much better than commercial meat products, still has an improper ratio of omega-6s to omega-3s, which is caused by the cattle being fed grain, a completely unnatural food source, even if organic!

   Grass-fed meat is best. Grass-fed cattle produce meat with much higher levels of the beneficial omega-3 fatty acids and lower levels of omega-6 fatty acids than grain-fed cattle. Grass-fed beef is also higher in beta-carotene, calcium, magnesium vitamin E, potassium and some B vitamins. It is also higher in beneficial conjugated linoleic acid (CLA), which is known to have anti-cancer properties.

2. Saturated fat is good for you! Eat meat with saturated fats—not lean meats. It is not the protein that we need in high amounts, rather it is protein combined with the saturated fat! Read the literature at *Weston A. Price Foundation* and decide for yourself (www.westonaprice.org/).

3. Eat smaller portions of meat. A simple rule of thumb for meat portion sizes is to eat a portion that fits into the palm of your hand and is no thicker than your middle finger. You can personally test for portion size to see if the palm-sized portion is a good rule for you to follow.

4. Eat organ meats like liver from time to time.

5. Avoid high temperature cooking. Stews, slow roasted meats, lightly sautéed food and soups are ideal.

6. Most prepared meats (i.e., sausages, etc.) contain toxins and preservatives. These additives are the culprits, which are then magnified by the unhealthy meat.

7. Avoid BBQ meats as much as possible. The charring creates carcinogens, which is not good for a prostate!

Just got to have BBQ'd meat? The smell is just too much for you? Well, here is an occasional compromise that can reduce the toxins. Just don't go overboard! It's the compounds called heterocyclic amines (HCA), which seem to be one of the culprits in prostate cancers, caused by cooking on the grill.

Well, a new study shows that marinating meat in special herbs sharply reduces the level of HCAs.

The researchers marinated steaks in three different types of marinade for an hour each, and then grilled them at 400 degrees, five minutes per side. They also grilled steaks minus the marinade. Amazingly, the steaks marinated in a "Caribbean mixture" containing thyme, red and black pepper, allspice, rosemary, and chives— showed an 88 percent reduction in HCAs. An herb marinade composed of oregano, basil, onion, jalapeno, parsley, and red pepper provided a 72 percent reduction, and a third marinade with paprika, red pepper, oregano, black pepper, garlic, and onion brought a 57 percent reduction.

Marinated Meats Less Toxic by J. Barron, tiny.cc/gn5yzw

You still must avoid flare-ups from burning fat because this is a whole other danger, so cook at the lowest temperatures that you can. BBQ for special occasions only, not regular use!

For an in-depth review of traditional and primitive diets from around the world as well as conclusions on saturated fats, meat, a balanced whole foods diet, and more, please read this these articles:

Ancient Dietary Wisdom for Tomorrow's Children (tiny.cc/xo5yzw)

Characteristics of Traditional Diets (tiny.cc/4p5yzw)

What's Wrong with "Politically Correct" Nutrition? (tiny.cc/8q5yzw)

For an in-depth look at meat, read this book: *Why Grass Fed Is Best! The Surprising Benefits of Grass Fed Meats, Eggs, and Dairy Products* (tiny.cc/cs5yzw)

Please read this article to fully understand the definitions of grass-fed and organic meat, as there are many caveats: *Ensure Your Organic Meat is Truly Organic* (tiny.cc/fu5yzw).

Dairy

If you want controversy, dairy is up there with fats and meat! Everyone has strong opinions on this, especially the holistic health specialists. Conventional nutritionists say dairy is an essential food. Many others blame dairy for what ails you, and they may be right!

The same sad story exists today around dairy as it does with meat and fats: the modern agricultural and processing methods and government regulations have transformed a once healthy food into a sickness-generating toxin.

The same bad practices plague dairy: modern feedlots, confined quarters, unnatural feed like grains, pesticide-ridden foods and hormone additives and antibiotics have all wreaked havoc on milk products and the consumers who eat it. Add pasteurization and homogenization—you have dairy foods that are now unfit for human consumption.

Sure you can eat it and may not be able to trace its effects, but over time the naysayers of dairy will prove to be right. Not because dairy products in and of themselves are unhealthy foods per se (as many pundits claim) but because of what we have done to these foods.

My take on dairy: Some people have evolved to have a family heritage of being able to digest dairy easily while others (e.g., often Asians) have troubles with it, especially the non-raw (pasteurized) varieties.

If you have not been eating dairy, go slow by first testing and often retesting (see Chapter 9) the different dairy products you choose. Most people who have had problems with dairy will find that raw versions are far less reactive and easier to tolerate. Many raw cheeses, butter and ghees have no lactose, which is a culprit—other than pasteurization—that may cause sensitivities/allergies in some people.

Milk and Pasteurization

Most milk today is ultra-pasteurized, even organic milk. Ultra-pasteurization is the process of heating milk to a temperature of at least 280°F, well above the 212°F boiling point. This is done to give milk a longer shelf life and to kill germs from the unsanitary growing conditions of cramped quarters for the cows.

What is less known is the effect that the ultra-pasteurization process has on the natural enzymes in the milk and consequently the effects this has on the human body. The *Weston A. Price Foundation* states:

> *Rapid heat treatments like pasteurization, and especially ultra-pasteurization, actually flatten the molecules so the enzymes cannot do their work. If such proteins pass into the bloodstream (a frequent occurrence in those suffering from 'leaky gut,' a condition that can be brought on by drinking processed commercial milk), the body perceives them as foreign proteins and mounts an immune response. That means a chronically overstressed immune system and much less energy available for growth and repair.*
>
> *Ultra-Pasteurized Milk by L. J. Forristal,* tiny.cc/0v5yzw

Not to mention the ill effects of milk packaging! Read from the same website about the dangers of this health destroying process and the risks of the plastic containers that are common today.

> *While the processing of [ultra high temperature processed] milk creates palatability problems and possible health risks, so does its packaging—both the aseptic boxes and plastic containers. For example, phthalates and other endocrine disrupting compounds (EDC) can leach into the milk.*
>
> *Ultra-Pasteurized Milk by L. J. Forristal,* tiny.cc/0v5yzw

The normal pasteurization process heats milk up to around 250°F and uses pressure as well. Perhaps it is a bit better than the ultra-pasteurized type, but still is not a healthy or whole food.

In *Timeless Secrets of Health and Rejuvenation*, Andreas Moritz also describes the problems with milk pasteurization:

Once milk is pasteurized, or ultra heat-treated, its natural enzyme population is destroyed. Yet the enzymes are needed to make the milk nutrients available to the body cells. **Newly born calves die within six months when fed with pasteurized cow's milk.** *One can only imagine the turmoil that must be going on in the tiny intestinal tract of a baby who is fed with pasteurized milk or sterilized milk formula. As mentioned before, such babies usually develop colic, bloated and chubby, discharge mucus, catch colds frequently, are restless, and cry a lot.*

Timeless Secrets of Health and Rejuvenation by A. Moritz, amzn.to/n71lG7

Organic, raw milk from grass-fed animals is the healthiest dairy. This is the dairy of yesteryear, and if milking and dairy facilities are meticulous and clean the food is completely safe and highly nutritious.

Raw milk has been proven to prevent scurvy, the flu, TB, and allergies. Pastured whole, raw milk contains essential fat soluble vitamins A, D and K2 along with B12, B6, C, calcium, iron, iodine and minerals which can easily be utilized by the body. When milk is pasteurized, most of these nutrients are destroyed. The remaining protein, calcium and D vitamins are denatured and poorly absorbed. In other cases, the body begins an attack on what it views as a foreign substance and allergic reactions can develop. Pasteurized milk consumption has been linked with osteoporosis, tooth decay, arthritis, heart disease and cancer.

High Quality Raw Milk Enhances Health while Pasteurized Milk Contributes to Illness by M. Goldstein, tiny.cc/505yzw

Read more at *What is Real Milk?* (tiny.cc/in6yzw)

Dairy Un-Forbidden: Discover the Virtues of Raw Milk (tiny.cc/wo6yzw)

I finally found some raw milk and was able to personally test it. Commercial milk and the best organic pasteurized milk that I can find—including yogurts of most brands—personally test NO for me, but the raw milk and the raw milk yogurt made at 180°F have a YES test result. In addition, when I consume raw milk my tongue does not have a white coating in the morning, which is a sign of poor digestion. Pasteurized milk causes a white coating on my tongue by morning.

I was also able to find some delicious raw milk cheeses at the health food store, so look for those and perhaps at extensive cheese counters in upscale supermarkets, as they may have some as well (especially Québec or French ones). I also tested YES for raw milk cheese while other pasteurized cheeses, including organic ones, are NOs for me.

In *Timeless Secrets of Health and Rejuvenation* (amzn.to/n71lG7), Moritz went on to describe how boiling milk can be beneficial. To differentiate, slowly boiling at a lower temperature of about 180° to 212°F, rather than a rapid heating under pressure to temperatures between 250° and 280°F for pasteurization are two completely different processes. The slow boiling at a lower temperature is something that traditional cultures have done for a long time.

Boiling fresh, non-pasteurized milk before consumption seems to have a beneficial effect. Milk protein begins to break down into amino acids during boiling, which makes it easier to digest and absorb. This may be one of the reasons why East Indians always boil their milk before use. They also know that milk has adverse effects when its fat is removed.

And just a note on digestibility and milk temperatures, in *Timeless Secrets of Health and Rejuvenation* (amzn.to/n71lG7), Moritz let us in on the life of enzymes and the ideal environment required for maximum digestion:

Cold milk is very difficult to digest. As the cold milk touches the warm stomach lining, the nerve endings of the stomach become 'numb' or insensitive, and its cells tighten or shrink. This inhibits the secretion of gastric juices, which is required to digest milk protein. The cold condition of the milk may even be responsible for leaving those proteins undigested that are known to cause allergic reactions. Enzymes require a specific temperature to be able to act on the food; if the temperature is too low the proteins will not be broken down properly, hence the intense irritation of the mucus lining.

While organic forms of dairy are far superior to the commercial ones, if they are pasteurized, as most are, then you still are not getting as ideal a food as raw grass-fed milk and dairy.

Important enzymes like lactase are destroyed during the pasteurization process, which causes many people to not be able to digest milk. Additionally, vitamins (such as A, C, B6 and B12) are diminished and fragile milk proteins are radically transformed from health nurturing to unnatural amino acid configurations that can actually worsen your health. The eradication of beneficial bacteria through the pasteurization process also ends up promoting pathogens rather than protecting you from them . . .

Once milk has been pasteurized its physical structure is changed in a way that can actually cause allergies and immune problems.

10 Lies and Misconceptions Spread by Mainstream Nutrition by Dr. Mercola, tiny.cc/fr6yzw

Homogenized milk is a process that prevents the fat content of the milk from separating. High pressure and more heat used during homogenization make the milk even harder to digest resulting in allergies in many people.

Raw milk and dairy are a completely natural wholesome food compared to all the other processed varieties—even organic. Suspend your judgment until you can test raw dairy!

For sources of raw milk and cheese, visit the site *Where Can I Find Real Milk?* (tiny.cc/jt6yzw). I also suggest you try raw goat or sheep milk and cheeses.

You can also find sources of raw milk in cow share programs, local farmers, and here at the *Raw Milk Institute* (tiny.cc/2u6yzw).

By the way, many of the arguments about the dangers of raw milk are completely false. Pasteurization came about because growers in NY in the early 1900s used such cramped quarters that the only way to deal with the unsanitary conditions was to advocate for pasteurization rather than provide safe sanitary conditions and happy cows.

Nuts and Seeds

These are wonderful healthy foods—but there's a catch! Just like grains and beans, nuts and seeds contain high levels of the anti-nutrient phytic acid, as well as enzyme inhibitors that cause unnoticed reactions to mild reactions all the way to severe allergic reactions in some people. This is in addition to the mineral binding effect that phytic acid has, thereby reducing mineral content in the body and prostate. (See *Anti-Nutrients* in Chapter 2.)

For me, it was the unnoticed response that gradually worsened in me. I used to eat lots of nuts and nut butters. After my prostate condition developed, I became more and more sensitive to nuts until I reached the point that I would end up blocked and no pee would come out! Cashews, almonds, pine nuts, Brazil nuts, walnuts, pecans and even sesame seeds shut me down at various times. No fun.

Now I know why: it was due to the phytates and the enzyme inhibitors. These natural components protect the nut from predators while growing and from sprouting prematurely. Nuts need to be phytate reduced to be healthy and easy to digest. Soaking overnight in warm water with some sea salt and then dehydrating in your oven at 125–150° will do the trick. This process also makes them even better tasting and crunchier. Soaking and then sprouting also works great.

If you only have occasional small amounts of nuts and seeds in your diet and you do not have any reactions and no prostate condition, you are probably okay and can eat nuts and seeds without phytate-reduction techniques in moderate quantities. However, if you regularly consume nuts, seeds or nut milks like almond milk, or nut or seed butters, then it would be best to make your own by soaking them first, or finding ones that are done for you—more and more available now in health food stores.

Nuts have many beneficial qualities for the prostate. Almonds are perhaps the easiest to digest, especially when soaked overnight and dried or roasted afterwards. Both walnuts and Brazil nuts can help reduce the size of the prostate and the growth of prostate cancer. Soak the nuts and dry them for optimum bioavailability and for phytate reduction.

Personally test all nuts to see if your body can handle them. A NO response before soaking and drying may turn into a YES after doing so. But even with a YES, it is best to incorporate soaking if you want the most benefit with the least amount of reaction. Beware of almonds that are not organic, as California almonds are now sprayed and walnuts irradiated. Personally test for how many nuts to eat daily if you are sensitive to them. Do not overeat nuts.

Avoid cracked nuts, as they can go rancid easily. Watch out for nut butters as they easily cause adverse reactions. Avoid mixed nuts and dried fruit. Certainly avoid canned, packed and processed commercial nuts.

Pumpkin seeds have high levels of phytic acid and need to be soaked. While many health advocates claim benefits for the prostate in eating pumpkin seeds and pumpkin butter because of the zinc content, but unless the phytic acid is reduced by soaking, regular consumption of pumpkin seeds will be more harmful than beneficial.

Sesame seeds have very high phytic acid levels, and this is one food where the hull is best removed. (Traditional cultures all removed them.) It is best if you buy white—not unhulled brown—sesame seeds.

I used to eat lots of sesame seeds, mostly with the hull on the seed. I ate sesame butter, gomasio (roasted sesame seeds with salt), ground seeds in smoothies and plain seeds cooked with rice. One night after having some sesame seeds, I had a reaction in my prostate; the seeds had caused a block in my pee tube . . . and misery. The next morning I personally tested everything I had eaten and discovered the culprit—sesame seeds!

Tahini is hull-less and, therefore, a good sesame seed product whereas sesame butter found in health food stores is made with sesame seeds with the hulls on (and lots of phytates)—avoid sesame butter.

There are many other wonderful seeds like chia and flax seeds, both known as superfoods, but I have had reactions to them, perhaps by eating too many. Moderation, even with beneficial seeds and nuts, is essential. Reduction of the toxins by soaking is highly recommended.

To read more on the high nutrient content of nuts and seeds, visit the website for *The World's Healthiest Foods* (www.whfoods.com/).

Fruits and Vegetables

The best advice is to eat a wide variety of fruits and vegetables, while paying attention to seasonality and locality for your choices—these foods are more vital and have more nutrients because they are harvested closer to full ripeness.

It is especially important to personally test (see Chapter 9) to see whether foods from the tropics are suitable in mid-winter in northern locales. Tropical fruits are not ideal foods for daily use in our temperate climates, especially in winter.

The healthier you are, the less will you experience reactions. You will be able to eat a wide variety of foods without problems. If you are in a more critical situation, testing becomes essential as your body rebuilds and doesn't yet have the strength to deal with less than ideal inputs.

I bet you didn't know this about sweet potatoes, the red-fleshed ones (nor did I):

> [They] ranked number one in nutrition out of all vegetables by the Center for Science in the Public Interest because they are such a rich source of dietary fiber, natural sugars, complex carbohydrates, protein, carotenoids, vitamin C, iron and calcium.
>
> Nine Reasons to Eat More Sweet Potatoes by E. Walling, tiny.cc/tx6yzw

When buying local produce, ensure it is organic and not sprayed. Read this article for a personal, environmental health perspective, *Local and Organic Food Farming: Here's the Gold Standard* (tiny.cc/ry6yzw).

Learn to Read Labels on Produce

You will see a series of numbers on produce like an orange, usually 5 numbers in a row (e.g., 94046). The first number is the key to knowing how it was grown:

#9 =	Organic (selenium and nutrient rich)
#8 =	GMO foods (genetically modified genes and enzymes, also containing pesticides and herbicides)
#4 =	Conventional produce (contains pesticides and herbicides)

Eat a wide variety of fruits and vegetables both raw and cooked every day; this includes lacto-fermented raw foods. Decide the proportion of raw foods in your diet based on where you live, the current season, your sunlight exposure on your skin, the current strength of your digestive tract (cooked is better for most foods if you have compromised digestion as most of us do), your sensitivity to particular foods and the results you receive when you personally test (see Chapter 9).

Do not assume that you can eat all vegetables or fruits because they are natural. If you have a health condition, you can have unknown reactions or slow weakening from many of them. This was such a surprise for me to learn that even my own garden grown kale or beet leaves caused reactions sometimes!

See the Farmigo website to find produce growers in your area (www.farmigo.com). This Mercola website offers information on local growers, too (tiny.cc/316yzw).

Nightshade Vegetables

Potatoes, tomatoes, eggplants and bell peppers are part of the nightshade group of vegetables. Sensitive eaters may have reactions to some of these vegetables, including prostate reactions, arthritis and rheumatism, nervous system reactions and more.

These vegetables contain harmful glycoalkaloids. Green parts of potatoes and their eyes have high amounts of these toxins. Many people are unknowingly allergic to tomatoes. The solanine in these foods can be harmful. It is best to test nightshades often and to stop their use entirely if you react, at least for some time period.

And it is best to consume your potatoes with butter to help digest them properly.

Oxalate Vegetables

Chives, beet leaves, Swiss chard, rhubarb, spinach and parsley contain high quantities of oxalic acid. Oxalic acid binds with minerals like calcium and iron, forming urinary stones, which can easily irritate the prostate. Oxalate vegetables should only be eaten on occasion and only if you personally test positive for them.

Sweeteners

Sugars are associated with the growth of cancer cells because sugar is food for cancer cells. This includes cancer of the prostate. Sugars create digestion problems and obesity especially when combined with refined white carbs.

Sugar consumption has increased drastically. Our ancestors ate at most one tablespoon per day of natural unprocessed sugars; today we consume a cup or more per day on average, and mostly of the highly refined varieties like white sugar or worse—the high fructose corn syrup! Imagine those at the high end of the scale eating way more than the average.

Sugar is found now in most prepared foods. High fructose corn syrup, a highly refined sweetener, is even more deadly than sugar cane. See this article for more information: *The Murky World of High-Fructose Corn Syrup* (tiny.cc/336yzw).

Fructose and high fructose corn syrup (HFCS), found in many fast foods and processed foods, are deadly sweeteners linked to metabolic syndrome, diabetes, cardiovascular disease and obesity. See this article for more information: *Diabetes, Obesity and Metabolism Journal Article* (tiny.cc/a56yzw).

Also see Dr. Robert Lustig's YouTube video, *Sugar: The Bitter Truth*, that explains the damage caused by fructose (tiny.cc/g66yzw). Fructose is one of the primary causes of obesity.

Another danger now with high fructose corn syrup found in so many supermarket foods, fast foods, soda pop and more—is the reality that most of the corn grown to make the syrup is made from GMO corn. Genetically engineered foods have made terrible cancerous lesions in rats in a recent big study out of France (see the section on toxins in Chapter 2).

Avoid fruit juices, as their fructose is worse than regular sugar. A can of orange juice has as much sugar content as a can of Coke. If you must have fruit juices then dilute them with water 4:1—that's 4 units of water to 1 unit of juice, not the opposite!

Artificial sweeteners are no better. People use them in the hope that the artificial sweeteners are less harmful and because of the lack of calories. They actually increase your sugar cravings. And the chemicals are alien to your body and actually cause weight gain! You are just trading in one bad habit for a worse one. Read all about the dangers of artificial sweeteners at *Sugar-Free Blues* (tiny.cc/o76yzw).

Healthy Sugar Alternatives

- Real maple syrup (not imitation)—the darker it is the more nutrients in maple syrup. Choose grade B or C, or #2 or #3 (different grading systems). Maple syrup contains potassium and calcium as well as nutritionally significant amounts of zinc and manganese. Zinc is a crucial prostate mineral. In moderation, rich, dark, organic, pure maple syrup is your sweetener of choice. If you can't find it in your local health food store, you can find some at this website: tiny.cc/vkyus
- Raw, unfiltered honey—the darker the better as, like maple syrup, darker honey has more trace elements. (Cooking honey destroys its healthy enzymes. So use only in non-cooking recipes.)

- Molasses
- Dehydrated sugar cane juice, sold as Sucanat (tiny.cc/k2uq8) and Rapadura (tiny.cc/lrq1c)
- Date sugar
- Organic Coconut Sugar (tiny.cc/i915v)
- Consume your sweeteners and desserts in moderation! One to two tablespoons maximum per day is more than enough.

Water

Our most essential "food" after air—water—heals or harms. If you haven't been paying attention to the quality of the water you drink and consume in beverages and cooking, start immediately!

In most cities, tap waters contain chlorine, fluoride and residues of all kind of toxic chemicals. Often tap water is not fit for human consumption. Bottled waters are not much better.

> *The majority of bottled water on the market is no different than basic tap water. It does, however, cost 50–100 times more per gallon than basic tap. Even worse, if the water is bottled in plastic it leaches xenoestrogenic chemicals into the water. These chemicals disrupt the hormonal balance that should be present in the body. An example is bisphenol A (BPA), which is linked to neurodevelopmental problems in children. BPA can stimulate premature puberty and even lead to breast development in males. BPA has also been linked to breast, uterine, ovarian, and prostate cancers.*
>
> *Bottled Water is Hazardous to You and Our World by Dr. D. Jockers,* tiny.cc/5h7yzw

The simplest solution is to use a water purifier. There are many options here. A countertop unit like Brita will remove chlorine but not much else. Aquasana makes highly rated and affordable filters that you can use at the sink or for the whole house (bit.ly/peKByu).

I prefer a water distiller. Some health pundits claim distilled water robs your body of minerals. Water contains very small amounts of minerals in general. Get them from your food! I sometimes add a quarter teaspoon of sea salt to the distilled water per gallon to add a touch of minerals back and to revitalize the water.

I prefer distillers that have a stainless steel chamber and a glass collection bottle, not a plastic one. I use Waterwise's smallest unit: the Waterwise 4000 (tiny.cc/ok7yzw). This distiller is made in the U.S. and distills a gallon in about 3–4 hours. You will also find them on Amazon, but be wary of plastic ones (tiny.cc/7lvc1).

Berkey Water Filters is another highly rated water filter with many sizes for home and traveling (tiny.cc/xm7yzw).

An inexpensive way to get rid of most chlorine in water for bathing is to use vitamin C. Add 1–2 grams of vitamin C powder in your bath water (tiny.cc/un7yzw). This is particularly useful if you want to lie in the bathtub without suffering the irritating effects of chlorine.

We absorb chlorine and heavy metals from the water when we bathe and shower—lots of it. Over time you are adding greatly to your toxic load. You can get simple inexpensive devices that you can put in your bath water or showerhead, or filter all of your home's water. Check these items out at Amazon to find something that suits your needs and budget:

Bath Dechlorinators (tiny.cc/xd3vp)

Whole House Chlorine Water Filters (tiny.cc/1n41c)

Here is a simple, inexpensive and highly effective showerhead from Waterwise (tiny.cc/pxk9tw). This is what they say:

> *Showerwise reduces inhalation of vapors and the absorption of chemicals by effectively removing chlorine and reducing contaminants including iron, lead, arsenic, mercury, and hydrogen sulfide. Your body can absorb more in a ten minute shower than from drinking the same water all day!*
>
> *Showerwise also controls several types of bacteria including algae, fungi and mold.*
>
> *Deluxe Showerwise Shower Filtration System by Waterwise, tiny.cc/uu7yzw*

The bottom line on water is to personally test it to see that what you are using is best for you. If you are unsure of what type of filter system may be better, see if you can find someone who has a machine and personally test their water. When traveling I just test the bottled waters in the supermarkets to see what is best and distilled wins for me each time.

How Much Water Should You Drink?

Most health advocates say we should drink at least 8 cups of water a day (8 oz. per cup). They say that most people are chronically dehydrated and need more water to vitalize all the internal organs. Since our bodies are 70% water, they say it is essential to drink enough.

While it may be true that we are dehydrated, that may have to do with our improper diets of too much of the wrong foods, laden with excess commercial salt and too many toxins. I believe that is the first place to make changes.

The recommended notion then is to flush the toxins out with water, but that may be adding to the problem:

> *If you are drinking lots of water throughout the day, your stomach acid will become diluted, leading to acid reflux and all the other problems herein described. In addition, too much water may cause mineral depletion and imbalances, which can further contribute to digestive disorders.*
>
> *Paradoxically, over-consumption of water may also cause constipation. When too much water is added to a high-fiber diet, the fibrous foods swell and ferment in the intestinal tract, leading to gas, bloating and other uncomfortable digestive symptoms. This expanded mass may be too large to pass easily.*

So as people succumb to drinking large quantities of water, not only will they lower the acid levels in the stomach, their digestion and nutrient absorption will be compromised. Over time this also contributes to malnourishment.

Acid Reflux: A Red Flag by K. Pirtle, tiny.cc/tk8yzw

Roger Mason in *Zen Macrobiotics for Americans* describes a very similar viewpoint. While there are parts of his book I no longer agree with, this does make sense to me:

It is surprising to many people to learn that we should only drink when we are thirsty. We should only drink when we feel the need to drink, when we have a true thirst. We never have a false thirst for water like we have a false thirst for food. Many dietary advocates advise drinking literally quarts of water per day whether you are thirsty or not. These people claim we're 'dehydrated'. Don't listen to this. This drink-as-much-as-you-can theory is very harmful—'drink eight glasses a day'.

The proponents go on the theory you can flush your kidneys out like sewer pipes. Quite the opposite is true in that the more you drink the less efficiently your kidneys operate. Your kidneys are not like the plumbing system in your house. Kidneys filter, absorb, and diffuse, and thus should not be overloaded with water they don't want nor need. Drinking too much liquids overworks your kidneys so they can't do what they are designed to do. When you take in too much water the cells close up and unfiltered water is diverted to the large intestine in desperation. The water then goes to the bladder to be passed out without removing the toxins from your system. The toxins are therefore left in your body.

ONLY DRINK WHEN THIRSTY and don't drink if you are not thirsty. Your urine should never be cloudy but rather clear with a deep yellow color to show that lots of toxins are contained in it. It is very difficult to drink when you're not thirsty. This goes against our very instincts when we drink if we don't need to.

Zen Macrobiotics for Americans by R. Mason, amzn.to/rtgETB

Many of the gurus on water and health fail to adjust for climate, age, body size, activity level, etc. It seems everyone copies everyone's recommendations, and we are convinced we need our 8 glasses minimum! See how many people carry around water bottles drinking constantly, blindly following these dictates.

A recent study at CBC has now debunked the crazy excess water drinking myth (tiny.cc/x68yzw).

Some pundits claim you should never drink during meals. Sipping small amounts of water *if you are thirsty* actually helps digestion. Also, it's best not to drink lots 15–20 minutes before and after eating so as not to dilute the digestive juices. And avoid cold water. That is harmful to the kidneys and what affects the kidneys will impact your prostate. In the East, they never drink cold water—always warm.

My take on water is to drink only when thirsty and err a bit on the side of extra rather than too little because being dehydrated will make you lethargic and tired. Just monitor your urine color, which should have a clear, light yellow color. I also like hot water with some fresh lemon squeezed in with a little honey or maple syrup, especially first thing in the morning. It helps the liver get ready for the day's jobs!

Caffeinated Drinks

You will find lots of information both for and against caffeinated drinks, especially around coffee. Some researchers say caffeine is very healthy and others say just the opposite. A simple solution is to personally test the caffeinated drinks that you regularly consume. You will know right away. If you get a YES, then do not assume it means that you can drink as much as you want. Test again to find your optimum number of cups (see *Personal Testing* in Chapter 9).

Many people recommend green tea for its health benefits. Test that to see if it is okay for you and see if decaf green varieties are better. Always choose organic versions.

Teas and Herbal Teas

You will find that many herbal teas can be troublesome for your prostate if you have a condition . . . so be careful and test often.

Beer Wine and Liquor

Fermented beers can be a wonderful beverage, especially from small homemade batches or microbreweries.

Try organic wines, as grapes are one of the most-sprayed foods. Personally test to see if you can drink wine, whether red or white, and how much.

Test any liquor you want. I find that there are some fine liquors I can drink a bit of on occasion without a reaction, but most times I get a NO response.

Lacto-Fermented Foods

Probiotics are live microorganisms in our foods and are proven to be beneficial to the digestive system. Probiotics improve the absorption of nutrients and promote a healthy immune system. This is a very important food group that helps digestion immensely.

It is the good bacteria and enzymes found in unpasteurized lacto-fermented foods like traditional yogurt, sauerkraut and pickles (without vinegars) that are not only tasty but also help prevent gas and irritable digestion, as well as many other benefits.

Today, many health gurus highly recommend adding all kinds of digestive enzymes in the form of supplements to your diet. There is also a trend to add enzymes like acidophilus in processed yogurts and other foods.

A far superior way to get probiotics is from traditional lacto-fermented foods. These foods have been used around the world in all cultures to preserve foods and to aid digestion. They do work wonders—I can vouch for that. The enzymes help digestion in the upper stomach where there are no digestive fluids and further aid digestion by providing lactic acid.

Lacto-fermented foods, such as natural yogurt, contain plentiful amounts of natural probiotics, which normalize the acidity of the stomach and do much more:

Like the fermentation of dairy products, preservation of vegetables and fruits by the process of lacto-fermentation has numerous advantages beyond those of simple preservation. The proliferation of lactobacilli in fermented vegetables enhances their digestibility and increases vitamin levels . . .

These beneficial organisms produce numerous helpful enzymes as well as antibiotic and anticarcinogenic substances. Their main by-product, lactic acid, not only keeps vegetables and fruits in a state of perfect preservation but also promotes the growth of healthy flora throughout the intestine.

Nourishing Traditions: The Cookbook that Challenges Politically Correct Nutrition and the Diet Dictocrats by S. Fallon and M. Enig, amzn.to/nB9irS

Here is another wonderful book filled with simple recipes to brew all kinds of delicious fermented treats:

Wild Fermentation: The Flavor, Nutrition, and Craft of Live-Culture Foods (tiny.cc/ma9yzw)

These lacto-fermented foods are great sources of probiotics and are ideal for daily eating at each meal—natural, unpasteurized versions without vinegars are the most potent:

- Yogurt
- Tamari
- Miso
- Tempeh
- Sauerkraut
- Buttermilk
- Kefir
- Cottage cheese
- Sourdough breads
- Pickles of all kinds

Use these natural forms of probiotics regularly and see the difference they make to your overall digestion. Always test first to ensure your compatibility, and start with very small amounts. Learn more about personal testing in Chapter 9.

Lacto-fermented beverages are ubiquitous in traditional cultures- from kefir beer in Africa to kvass and kombucha in Slavic regions. Lacto-fermented foods are artisanal products—instead of mass produced items preserved with vinegar and sugar—which taste delicious and confer many health benefits. They add valuable enzymes to the diet, and enhance digestibility and assimilation of everything we eat.

Nasty, Brutish and Short? by S. F. Morell, tiny.cc/xc9yzw

Read more about the benefits of probiotics here:

California Dairy Research Foundation: US Probiotiocs (tiny.cc/he9yzw)

National Center for Complementary and Alternative Medicine: Oral Probiotics (tiny.cc/qf9yzw)

You can get some wonderful cultured veggies at this site: www.culturedvegetables.net/.

Probiotic supplements are highly promoted, but the above foods are the best way to go. If you can't eat them because of travel or other reasons, then in the short term, taking probiotic supplements may be useful.

If you are coming off a bad diet, then both lacto-fermented foods and probiotics would be beneficial. Always personally test these lacto-fermented foods to know if they are right for you and what quantities you should have daily. Sometimes therapeutic doses of probiotics can help a leaky gut. Increase your intake for a short while by increasing your dose by a factor of 2–5 times per day.

Always test to ensure you are not overdoing it. Keep in mind that your body's needs do change! I had too much lacto-fermented sauerkraut it seems, because after a few months of eating sauerkraut at every meal I started to react. I tested, got a NO response, and realized again that even the best of the best can turn into its opposite with excess use. Seems like I am a slow learner! Thank goodness for being able to personally test foods!

Salt

Commercial salt—sodium chloride—may have the same chemical structure as sea salt, but there is a world of difference. The trace elements in sea salt, not found in commercial salt, are invaluable in providing needed minerals in our diets. For example, sea salt is high in zinc, the crucial prostate mineral. It is an easy switch to make from commercial salts. It will also save you from taking an inferior mineral supplement and from being harmed by commercial salt.

Just as with wine, there are many differences amongst the sea salts you can find today: from the thick slightly grayish Celtic Sea salts to the reddish/pinkish Himalayan and Utah salts from buried seas millions of years ago and to the pure, sun-dried Antarctic sea salts on the beaches of South West Africa to the wonderful Hawaiian ones and many, many more!

The pinkish color that some sea salts have comes from the trace minerals in the sea salt. These are ideal salts for your diet. You will find the taste far superior to bland commercial bleached and refined salt or—worse yet—the low-sodium salt substitutes that industry claims are better for you.

Some commercial salt has iodine added back in, but sea salt already contains that and many more nutrient minerals—60 to 80 other needed nutrients, in fact.

> *Part of the process for refined salt, or commercial table salt, involves the use of aluminum, ferro cyanide and bleach. These are all toxic materials that your body takes in with refined, commercial salt. And because of that process, almost all the vital minerals that real, unrefined sea salt can offer are removed! One or two servings of refined salt won't send you to the grave. But continued almost daily use will avail you to the perils of aluminum toxicity. Ferro cyanide is listed by the EPA as a toxic material for human consumption. You are probably aware of the hazards to human health of chlorine, which is used to bleach the salt.*

> *Why Himalayan Pink Crystal Salt is so Much Better for Your Health than Processed Table Salt by M. Adams, tiny.cc/4j9yzw*

Read this article to learn about the different perils of refined salt: *Confront Salt Confusion* (tiny.cc/ul9yzw).

Discover the world of sea salt. Try different varieties of sea salts to discover your favorite and to vary the micro mineral content. It is easy to find in any health store. You can also find sea salt at Amazon: tiny.cc/qefh4

Myth of Low Salt Diet

It has been drummed into our heads that a low salt diet is best for our health and our hearts. Here are 3 good articles to destroy that myth. Just make sure you eat high quality sea salt.

The Salt of the Earth (tiny.cc/5y9yzw)

Salt and Our Health (tiny.cc/9z9yzw)

Scant Evidence (tiny.cc/c19yzw)

Herbs and Spices

These items add great variety and flavor to our foods. The problem is that many can be irritants, especially if they are used frequently or if they have become stale. The only way to know is to personally test them from time to time. Another danger is that people often keep them around too long; they lose their freshness and can go off, which causes even further reactions. A year is about the maximum time to keep herbs and spices unless refrigerated.

I have had severe reactions to many herbs and spices thinking they are used in such small amounts that it wouldn't matter. Then I wisened up (I am slow sometimes!) and started testing them. Eat safe. Check 'em out!

Air

I call air a food because 10 to 20 times per minute we are consuming air. If the air is polluted you are at a health disadvantage. Make sure your home and car are protected if you live in air-polluted cities. Air purifiers with a negative ion generator can make a big difference. Read more at this site filled with expertise: *Office and Home Air Purifiers* (www.airpurifiers.com/).

How and When to Eat

Food is crucial for nourishing us. We need to learn to take more time than we are used to when it comes to preparing and eating whole foods. Food is your daily medicine and eating in a non-rushed manner is a good habit to develop.

Chewing more thoroughly than we are used to helps make the food much more digestible, so that we benefit from the high quality food choices we are now investing in.

In the Ayurvedic tradition, there are times that are thought best to eat that correspond with natural body biorhythms that enhance digestion. Those times are 8 am for breakfast, 12 noon for lunch and 6 pm for supper. Eating around these times (plus or minus an hour) is ideal and avoid eating after 8 pm, as our digestive juices decline rapidly in the evening.

Get With It!

Adjust to the fact that quality food will cost more than cheapo foods that harm you. What price is your health? Are new technological and electronic devices more desirable than great health? Find ways to make your health the top of your priority list because without good health, your quality of life will be impacted greatly.

You can still save by buying in bulk, joining food coops and buying clubs, buying direct from the grower, attending local farmers markets and starting to grow your own food, even on a balcony. Take a look at *Journey to Forever*'s website that has lots of resources for container gardening (tiny.cc/x39yzw).

And now you can get all kinds of healthy foods delivered to your door inexpensively anywhere in the U.S. Check out:

The *Green Polka Dot Box* (wwwyourgoodhealth.gpdb.com/)

It is a membership site that grows by referral. The benefits are truly amazing:

- Wholesale or deep discount pricing
- Free FedEx delivery
- Huge selection and major brands of organic foods
- Refrigerated, frozen and soon fresh organic veggies
- Personal care and Household
- Pet and Garden
- Supplements and natural remedies

Conclusion

- Eat widely across all food groups.
- Eat lacto-fermented foods to help you digest more.
- Eat slowly and chew well.
- If you want to drink while eating, sip rather than drink large quantities to aid your digestion.
- Limit desserts to one meal a day at most to lessen your addictions to sweets.
- Enjoy the rich tastes of natural wholesome foods!

Chapter 7: Superfoods

Superfoods are a group of foods that contain extra high amounts of beneficial nutrients. The list is subjective, as there is no official definition of what is and is not a superfood. Keep in mind, what may be a superfood for one could be harmful to another. The only way to know is to personally test each food you eat. That said, check some of these out: ghee, avocados and avocado oil, coconut oil, sauerkraut, miso, lemons and green superfoods.

Ghee

Ghee, also known as clarified butter, ideally made from the butter that comes from grass-fed cows, is a wonderful superfood. Ghee has a sweet buttery taste that adds both richness and flavor to your food. Ghee is basically butter with the milk protein and lactose taken out, leaving pure butter fat. Ghee has a higher burning point than butter, meaning you can cook it at much higher temperatures than butter without it burning. It's a great cooking oil.

Try some from Pure Indian Foods (www.pureindianfoods.com/).

They have several flavors, but I suggest you start with the plain version first.

Avocados and Avocado Oil

Avocados are a superfood delight and so delicious. They are filled with good fats that provide excellent anti-inflammatory benefits. Avocados contain:

- Phytosterols, including beta-sitosterol (found in Saw Palmetto)
- Carotenoid antioxidants
- Vitamins C and E
- Manganese
- Selenium
- Zinc
- Omega-3 fatty acids

Read more about avocados at tiny.cc/j79yzw

Avocado oil has a very high burning point, so it is great for cooking and is delicious on salads. Get extra virgin, cold-pressed, organic varieties. It will cost more but Avocado oil is a superb, versatile, very healthy oil for more moderate use (tiny.cc/ajyjo).

Want a potato chip made with healthy oils? Try these super yummy chips made with organic avocado oil: Avocado Chilean Lime Chips by Good Health (amzn.to/qehS7L).

As with all foods, remember not to overdo this oil. Since avocados are a tropical fruit, they are best eaten in moderation especially in winter if you test yes (see Chapter 9).

Coconut oil

This amazing oil, which is a saturated fat, is best in its extra virgin state. This means that like extra virgin olive oil, it has received the least amount of heat processing in order to preserve its optimum nutrient values. Coconut oil is perfect to cook with and to use in salads. It is also wonderful on your skin and hair. Read more here:

Latest Studies on Coconut Oil (tiny.cc/gaazzw)

Latest Headlines on Coconut Health (tiny.cc/hcazzw)

The Many Benefits of Coconut Oil and Coconut Butter (tiny.cc/edazzw)

> *Coconut oil also helps to balance hormones, stabilize blood sugar levels and boost the cellular healing process. It is also known to stimulate the thyroid and reduce stress on the liver and pancreas. This increases metabolism which helps us burn fat far more effectively while stimulating clean sources of energy that make us feel terrific.*

> *Make Sure You Consume Enough of this Super Food by Dr. D. Jockers,* tiny.cc/meazzw

Coconut oil also provides effective and natural sun protection without having to use toxic chemicals in conventional sun block. Coconut oil guards against free radicals, providing added protection against skin cancer. Mix coconut oil with African Shea butter and aloe vera for a simple and harmless sun protection formula. This combination is also wonderful as a moisturizer for your skin and hair.

Coconut water kefir is a fermented beverage especially beneficial for gut problems such as candida overgrowth. This drink is hard to find but easy to make. Visit tiny.cc/7fazzw for tips. Coconut water is also an excellent drink to use during fasting because of its high nutritional content.

One caveat: coconut is tropical and some sensitive people may not tolerate much coconut oil or other coconut products. I am one of those. As always, test to know.

Miso

A traditional oriental food, miso is a lacto-fermented food packed with great taste and benefits. Traditionally, miso is aged 6 months to 2 years. If you go to Japanese restaurants, then you must be familiar with miso soup.

Unfortunately modern Japanese miso is now adulterated from its past traditional greatness, often highly processed and containing MSG. It is best to buy organic versions free from GMO soybeans and MSG.

> *Many studies have shown the health benefits of miso on humans and animals. Benefits include reduced risks of breast, lung, **prostate,** and colon cancer, and protection from radiation.*

Miso has a very alkalizing effect on the body and strengthens the immune system to combat infection. Its high antioxidant activity gives it anti-aging properties.

Miso Soup: A Delicious Bowl Full of Health and Anti-Aging Benefits by B. Minton, tiny.cc/chazzw

Miso often is made with rice or barley added to the soybeans during the fermentation process. I find the rice version (genmai miso) mild and delicious. You can find some organic miso at this site: tiny.cc/0uqbt

Here is a very quick and simple way to use miso. Boil water, pour into a cup, add a teaspoon or more of miso and stir to dissolve. That's it—now you have a refreshing and uplifting drink with amazing health benefits.

Sauerkraut

This time-honored food, already talked about earlier, made from raw ingredients and salt is so beneficial for digestion. It can be an acquired taste for some people, so start slow with a small amount and use a young version rather than a longer-aged one.

Avoid pasteurized sauerkraut, as the pasteurization process destroys the beneficial nutrients in this superfood. Daily use will do wonders to your gut, so it is worth acquiring the taste. Start making your own since it is quick and easy to do. Here are some recipes for making your own sauerkraut and many more as *Nourishing Traditions* is THE cookbook to own: amzn.to/nB9irS

Start with only a small teaspoon of sauerkraut and increase the amount slowly to limit reactions in sensitive people.

Lemons (and Limes)

Lemons contain vitamin C and bioflavonoids, plant derivatives with antioxidant and anti-inflammatory—as well as anti-cancer—properties. Lemons are a superb food for the prostate.

High in potassium, lemons affect the body's biochemistry and pH levels in a positive and powerful way. Astringent in nature, lemons have an overall alkalizing effect on the body, even though they are acidic before entering the body.

I like to use a little lemon juice in place of vinegar in salad dressings. You can add it to steamed veggies, soups, sauces, dips and even desserts. I add a bit when making applesauce.

Some mornings I start the day with some lemon squeezed into a cup of very hot water and mixed with a teaspoon of honey. Use unpasteurized honey. According to Ayurvedic practices, this drink is good for the liver and aids digestion and the immune system. I also switch honey for maple syrup for variety. Read more about lemons and limes at this site: tiny.cc/hlazzw

Green Superfoods

Greens or green superfoods are highly promoted as powders, juices and supplements. These include wheatgrass, chlorella, blue-green algae, barley greens, parsley powders, spirulina and more. Packed with natural nutrients, vitamins and minerals, green superfoods come highly recommended by many practitioners. I won't get into all the claims here because, in the final analysis, you will be the judge by personally testing to see if green superfoods are right for you.

Remember—it is what you can digest that counts not what the profile is of the food. Greens are raw foods and can be difficult to process.

Be careful with these greens, they can cause reactions in you and your prostate. If greens test positive for you, they can be beneficial in helping you rebuild after years of poor diet habits because of their high nutrient content. You can read more here:

Natural News Store: search for "Green Superfoods" (bit.ly/qyNW4k)

Green Superfoods at Amazon (tiny.cc/afu5f)

Pure Synergy® Superfood is a top-of-the-line green product I used to take. There is quite the story of where and how it is made (tiny.cc/aoazzw).

It may be best to take a single green product rather than a mixture of many. You could test positive for an individual product, but a combination product could have something in it that disagrees with your system. So go to a health food store and start with single items to test. Then continue to test over time to ensure you do not end up with a negative reaction.

The simplest green product of all is liquid chlorophyll, particularly the brand World Organic Chlorophyll Liquid. It is the only green one that I have been able to tolerate well, perhaps because of its simplicity and compatibility with human blood (tiny.cc/tpazzw).

Greens may be useful as part of a cleansing diet for the short term and not every day use. Over the long term, I would bet that most people will eventually test NO to them. So be careful.

The best green superfood of all may in fact be raw milk! That way you let the cow do the hard work of digesting the greens, something they are optimally designed to do. It is now my preferred way to have my greens because I test NO for almost all of them and always YES for raw milk and yogurt.

Other Superfoods

Many people have their own lists of foods that contain high concentrations of valuable nutrients. Superfoods are a far superior way to get a vitamin or mineral that you think you may be missing rather than taking a supplement. I will list some here:

- Cod Liver Oil is such an important food source. It is a potent food with vitamin D and omega-3s in an easy to absorb form that makes it so potent (bit.ly/py6nHA).
- Manuka Honey—there has been lots of research on honey products. This is medicinal honey (tiny.cc/git1i).

- Swedish Bitters to balance all the tastes (tiny.cc/ayv3j).
- Evening Primrose Oil (tiny.cc/z2p6i), Black Currant Oil (tiny.cc/z8u0x) and Borage Oil (tiny.cc/cbjfo) are special, potent oils for very occasional use. Gamma Linoleic Acid (GLA), found in these oils, is an immune stimulator and anti-inflammatory
- Kelp has a high mineral content, especially iodine, which many people are deficient in. You can find powdered kelp with sea salt as a condiment that is quite tasty (tiny.cc/99om2).
- Wheat Germ Oil is an excellent source of natural vitamin E that can be added to smoothies (tiny.cc/nw1vh).
- Sprouts can be a powerhouse of concentrated nutrition. Soaking and then sprouting releases nutrients and decreases anti-nutrients like phytic acid in grains, nuts, beans and seeds. Sprouts are a great way of having fresh greens in the winter, bioavailable vitamins, minerals, amino acids, proteins, beneficial enzymes and phytochemicals. The only caveat is that you personally test them to ensure their compatibility as with any superfoods you eat. Sprouting is easy to do right in your kitchen. Get seeds at your local health food store or at Amazon: tiny.cc/h64gb.

Super Seeds

Seeds have healthy omega-3 fats and have minerals and vitamins our bodies need. Personally test these seed types before eating them, and then find the correct quantity. Often the best way to eat seeds is by grinding them first. I grind mine in a coffee grinder.

Chia Seeds

Organic chia seeds contain 15 times more magnesium than broccoli, 6 times more calcium than whole milk, 3 times more antioxidants than fresh blueberries, more fiber than flaxseed, plus more protein than soy and are extremely high in omega-3 fatty acids (tiny.cc/8v3sf).

As with other seeds and nuts, to reduce phytates you may need to sprout and then dry the seeds before consuming them. You can find some organic varieties made from sprouted seeds. I still test negative for chia, perhaps because I used too much before I knew about personally testing foods and phytates. If you get a YES response when you test, remember to go slow to start.

Flaxseeds

Touted today by many as a superfood, flaxseeds can be highly beneficial, as can the oil because of its beneficial high omega 3s. Best to take flax fresh grounded in your coffee grinder. If you use flax oil, it must be refrigerated to keep its potency. Add a teaspoon to your salads (tiny.cc/1twsl).

Pumpkin Seeds

Pumpkin seeds have been used in many cultures to treat BPH and prostatitis. They may also help cure prostate cancer. Pumpkin seeds are rich in zinc, a mineral for prostate health.

Pumpkin seeds and their oil may be useful, but pumpkin seeds do contain phytates, so it is best to buy them whole and soak the seeds to reduce the phytic acid before eating them (tiny.cc/luous).

Pumpkin seeds are also available as nut butter; I used to eat it often before I knew about the phytate anti-nutrient and had to stop when I had prostate reactions. I still test negative to pumpkin seeds, including its oil. So you know what to do now! Test for yourself to see if these seeds are good for you! (See *Personal Testing* in Chapter 9).

Antioxidants

This is a controversial subject with many health advocates proclaiming the benefits of taking antioxidants daily as a supplement. Although, some recent research suggests that over-indulging in antioxidants can have a harmful effect, this study refutes that claim: *Study Citing Antioxidant Vitamin Risks Based on Flawed Methodology, Experts Argue* (tiny.cc/70azzw).

The National Institutes of Health stated, "Antioxidants are substances that may prevent potentially disease-producing cell damage that can result from natural bodily processes and from exposure to certain chemicals." (tiny.cc/n2azzw)

Here is a summary of the supposed benefits of antioxidants:

Studies over the last 20 years have shown that free radical fighters found in a certain group of nutrients, namely antioxidants, can protect against a great many free radical initiated diseases. Antioxidants extinguish free radicals!

Free Radicals cause oxidation in the blood. Once oxidation occurs, disease can result. Antioxidants keep free radicals from causing oxidation in the blood, thus neutralizing disease. Also, stress, chemical pollution, environmental pollution, and the normal aging process increase the demands put upon the immune system.

Studies indicate antioxidants do more than protect against free radicals; they also stimulate the immune system's response to help fight existing diseases.

Antioxidant Benefits and Antioxidant Formulas by Health and Nutrition, tiny.cc/v3azzw

The article—*The Vital Role of Antioxidants in Achieving Optimum Health and Longevity*—lays out the specific ones that the author believes are the best (Acai, resveratrol, quercetin, pine tree bark, curcumin, lutein, zeaxanthin, lycopene, selenium, catalase, R-lipoic and humic/fulvic acid): tiny.cc/p6azzw

Another antioxidant of note is grape seed extract. A 2011 study discovered that grape seed extract could reduce men's risk of prostate cancer by 40–60%. The extract also has a positive impact on heart diseases. No studies have confirmed this yet (tiny.cc/n7azzw).

The realization is that all fresh foods contain lots of antioxidants and, if you are eating well, you are getting plenty of them, especially if you include some of the above-mentioned superfoods in your regular diet. That being said, some of you might want to add antioxidants to your daily regime.

I would suggest foods as your primary source, superfoods next, followed by food-based antioxidant supplements. My best advice is—again and again—to personally test before consuming them. I have found that most recommended antioxidants have a NO test result for me or—at best—test YES for a very short time, which saves me a lot of money. I must be getting what I need from my good diet—and so can you!

Cravings

I've told you about the conditions that create prostate disease, what you need to stop doing and what you need to start doing. One obstacle that often lies in the path of making these types of major lifestyle changes are cravings.

Cravings have many causes. A deficiency in a vital nutrient will easily urge you to crave certain foods. Unfortunately we end up binging on foods that only add to the problem. If you are missing enough good quality salt or saturated fats, for example, you could end up eating more and more devitalized breads, cookies and cakes—all of which will add weight and make you less healthy.

Although difficult to digest unless the grain is soaked first, gluten actually leads to cravings. This is because grain products like bread and muffins often contain gluten and produce pleasant feelings and the desire for more. If you have candida and parasites in your gut, then those lead to sugar and starch cravings because sugar and starch are food for those overgrowths.

A lack of saturated fats easily leads to cravings. If you have enough high quality saturated fats, you'll have fewer cravings. We feel satisfied when we eat them, and the cravings stop. The poor quality vegetable fats found in processed and fast foods become addictive because our bodies are never truly satisfied by them. Our bodies crave real food, not food-like substances!

The more you eat sugary foods, the more you will crave. Today many of our manufactured foods also have food additives designed to increase cravings for that product, which cause us to become addicted little by little.

Counting calories makes no sense since so many low caloric foods (i.e., non-foods like artificial sugars) actually are some of the worst offenders. Eating the wrong kind of calories—cakes, cookies or drinks with artificial sugars—simply cause weight gain and a host of problems.

What's the solution to constant cravings and weight gain? Slowly, little by little, start reducing the foods on the STOP list. Eat nourishing real foods instead. You will stop overeating because you will finally get what your body really needs and craves.

Healthy foods will do the trick! Your cravings will disappear as will pounds and pounds of unwanted fat. The Prostate Health Diet has real side benefits: a much healthier you!

Conclusion

Remember, superfoods are highly nutritious foods and some of them should definitely be incorporated into your healthy diet. As you are introduced to new products, personally test whether they would benefit your body or have a negative effect. Just because they're "super" doesn't mean they are super for you!

Some people choose to incorporate superfoods into their diet and skip supplementing all together. In Chapter 8, I discuss the pros and cons of supplementing.

Chapter 8: Supplements for Prostate Health

By far the most important supplement is your daily food! I can't emphasize this enough. Making the right food choices is **the key to health**. Don't let yourself be fooled into thinking that you can make up for poor food choices with supplements.

The complexities and bioavailability of nutrients, enzymes, naturally occurring minerals in food, vitamins, trace minerals (as found in high quality sea salts) and antioxidants found in whole foods cannot be replicated in a laboratory making synthetic versions of these essential ingredients for life. Even natural supplements are a far second to the benefits of natural whole foods eaten daily.

In the short term, if you are unable to take proper care by eating well, then supplements may have a place. But in the long term, your personally-tested optimum diet is the secret to your health and the health of your prostate!

Over the years of my search, I took all kinds of supplements, all highly recommended for prostate health. I spent a fortune. Overall with tests, books and supplements, my monthly average was easily $1000 to $2000 (for 10 years!). Most to no avail. That does not mean that supplements will not be effective for you, but they are not the panacea they are often made out to be.

I have been unable to tolerate many recommended supplement products at different points in time. Many supplements even caused a reaction, and I had to stop them. The problem with many of the products is the use of too many herbs or ingredients as well as binders and fillers to make them into capsules or tabs and which cause me to react. The theory is that more is better. But sometimes too many herbs can cause an irritation.

Personally test products to see which ones are best for you. It is better to test individual herbs if possible. Look for simpler prostate formulations. Many of the products that I reacted to had great research and the highest quality ingredients (organic or wild). I had to stop taking them.

When you do choose to supplement your diet, here are my rules of the game:

- use bioavailable natural supplements made from whole foods and herbs.
  - use freeze-dried forms, tinctures, extracts, concentrated or low temperature dried forms, which are closest to the whole foods that we eat.
  - Supplement on a temporary basis, not in the long term unless it is a concentrated food like cod liver oil.
  - Choose organic ingredients whenever possible.
- Avoid synthetic versions found in most commercial grades sold by large mainstream retailers (pharmacies and supermarkets). The quality and digestibility of these are questionable at best and may contain toxins.
- Supplements have become a mega-billion-dollar industry. You can find a huge variety that claim benefits for your prostate and overall health. Supplements can have a varying:

- amount of active ingredients
- quality of ingredients
- organic or commercial sources
- natural or synthetic ingredients
- type of binders or fillers
- price

What to Choose

In order of importance, these are the supplements worth considering when adding supplements to your healthy diet.

Vitamin D

Vitamin D studies show how deficient most people are today in this essential vitamin. **By increasing the amount of vitamin D in your body, you reduce your cancer risk by 50% or more, including prostate cancer!** Vitamin D has many other health benefits. It is the single most important nutrient for your good health. If you are low in it, you are much more prone to a whole range of health conditions.

I urge you to become better informed about sun exposure and vitamin D because it is such an important issue for your health (see *Sunlight Exposure* in Chapter 2).

Here are the conservative views of the National Institutes of Health. You will learn more about vitamin D from them but, according to many new studies, their minimum doses are outdated: tiny.cc/qabzzw

> *The results of two studies published in the British Journal of Cancer and Journal of Clinical Oncology found people with higher levels of vitamin D—at the time they were diagnosed—were more likely to survive.*

> *Vitamin D New Cancer Hope by University of Leeds*, tiny.cc/qbbzzw

These articles should reinforce the benefits of moderate sun exposure and adequate vitamin D supplementation when not enough sun is available.

If sun exposure cannot happen because of winter cold, due to dark, cloudy days, or because you lack the time, then the best way to supplement is with food sources like sardines or potent cod liver oil (see next section).

Liposomal Vitamin D3 is another great super high quality alternative. It comes in a liquid and uses a high potency Liposomal delivery that contains true fat for better absorption. This is an excellent way to take your D. For more information, go to the *GI for Life* website (tiny.cc/tcbzzw).

The next best choice for vitamin D is natural vitamin D3 supplements, but this is nowhere near as good as the cod liver oil or the liposomal form.

When buying any vitamin D, make sure that you're getting Vitamin D3 (cholecalciferol), not D2, which is an inactive form of Vitamin D (tiny.cc/a3mtl). D2 is about 10 times less effective because it is difficult for the body to absorb and use. Vitamin D3 is fat-soluble, so it is best to take it with some fat or oily food. That's why cod liver oil is so effective!

I prefer 1000 IU capsules of cod liver oil because you can easily personally test how many to take and adjust easily the amount. I took natural D3 before I learned about the benefits of cod liver oil.

Cod Liver Oil

This amazing concentrated food source provides digestible fat-soluble vitamin D plus vitamin A as well as rich amounts of eicosapentaenoic acid (EPA) and docasahexaenoic acid (DHA).

> Cod liver oil is also rich in eicosapentaenoic acid (EPA) and docasahexaenoic acid (DHA). The body makes these fatty acids from omega-3 linolenic acid. EPA is as an important link in the chain of fatty acids that ultimately results in prostaglandins, localized tissue hormones while DHA is very important for the proper function of the brain and nervous system.
>
> Cod Liver Oil Basics and Recommendations by S. Fallon and M. Enig, tiny.cc/zhbzzw

Natural cod liver oil is one of the best supplements I have ever taken. I use it in the winter as I live about 300 miles north of Seattle where skies are often grey and overcast for 6 months or more of the year. I use Green Pastures Blue Ice Royal Capsules, which contain natural cod liver oil, fermented to increase its absorbability, and high-vitamin butter oil (bit.ly/njtFp8). Read more about the combination of fish and butter oils: tiny.cc/jjbzzw

It is crucial that you personally test for the optimum quantity you need, and retest regularly to see if the quantity changes, especially as the seasons come and go. I needed 8 capsules per day when I started out (daily recommended dose is 2) and then it reduced over a few weeks to 1–2 per day, and then to none.

Be aware that many varieties of cod liver oil are bleached, which destroys the benefits. Find a high quality one such as those I have recommended above, and ensure you personally test it.

Over-Supplementing

I followed the advice of many natural health practitioners and, as a result, I took a ton of natural supplements every day, sometimes as many as 30–35 different ones per day! In the end, I realized that I was getting worse, and it was costing an arm and a leg to boot! Now that I know how to personally test (see Chapter 9), I have dropped down to 1–2 supplements at most per day, sometimes none. All the other supplements keep giving me a NO test response, although they are the highest quality organic supplements that I could find, including all kinds of antioxidants, that have wonderfully convincing research.

I am not saying you should avoid supplements. You just need to personally test to ensure these supplements are useful for you right now.

I have spent lots of time in the health food store testing many supplements that were of interest. I get mostly NOs and only occasionally a YES. So save your funds by personal testing as much as possible and invest your money in the best foods you can afford. That way you will get the most bang for your buck.

Keep in mind that your body's needs and testing responses will be unique to you. Testing will help you avoid unnecessary supplements and the possible weakening effects of some supplements, no matter how fantastic the literature is on them.

I have had reactions (including complete prostate blockage) to the very best supplements. I never suspected that such abundantly "good" ingredients could do that until I started personally testing everything and realized I could not make any critical assumptions about the benefits of even the supposed best of the best.

If you are relatively healthy, you probably won't have negative reactions like I did. Yet, these products may still be a waste of your money unless you test them to see if they will benefit you.

Now I personally test everything and no longer suffer the difficult side effects that I did before I instituted this practice. In many cases, a supplement will only test YES for a short period, after which it becomes harmful to you. So with these caveats in place, I will list some possible excellent products for you to check out, ideally at your health food store before you actually buy them.

Vitamins and Minerals

The more I learn about vitamins and minerals, the more convinced I am that it is a mistake to take them in pill form. The best way to get plenty of vitamins is through good eating habits, using sea salt and supplementing with high quality cod liver oil. You will get more than enough vitamins that way.

Your prostate relies on a lot of high quality zinc, magnesium and selenium to stay healthy, and you ain't gettin' it in your Standard American Diet (SAD) of denatured foods!

A healthy prostate contains a higher level of zinc than any other organ in the body. Zinc seems to protect the prostate from prostate diseases by keeping hormone levels in balance. As a bonus, zinc also boosts the immune system by destroying free radicals and bacteria.

This does not mean that you should over-supplement with zinc, which needs to be balanced with some copper. The best way to get zinc is by eating foods rich in zinc like oysters (best), wild salmon, liver (also contains copper), wheat germ, Brazil nuts, egg yolks, sesame and pumpkin seeds, lamb, sea salt (not commercial salt), dark grades of maple syrup and very dark chocolate. Make sure the meat and eggs are from grass-fed animals, not factory-imprisoned, grain-fed animals.

In *Timeless Secrets of Health and Rejuvenation* (amzn.to/n71lG7), Andreas Moritz says that we do **not** need extra vitamins and that they could actually be harmful to our health:

> *Taking extra vitamins can be harmful if the body is unable to make use of them and is left with the additional burden of having to break them down and eliminate them . . . can lead to vitamin poisoning (vitaminosis) which damages the kidneys . . . it would be more healthful and efficient to cleanse the body from accumulated toxins, stored proteins in the blood vessel walls, and impeding gallstones from the liver.*

To avoid imbalance in one way or the other, you should obtain your antioxidants only from one source—food . . . ideally of organic origin, still contain[s] more than enough vitamins to supply the body many times over . . .

The common practice of producing food synthetically and making it 'healthier' by adding synthetically derived vitamins and minerals is at the root of many health problems afflicting both children and adults in the developed world.

Synthetically derived "nutrients" are foreign matter to both animals and humans alike.

Timeless Secrets of Health and Rejuvenation by A. Moritz, (amzn.to/n71lG7)

I share these views after being a supplement junkie who took recommended vitamins and minerals for years with no positive outcomes. I gave it my best shot for years, yet my prostate just kept getting worse!

There is a large difference between the vitamins found in foods and many of the vitamins sold in pill form in our health food stores and drugstores. Vitamins in foods come with many cofactors—such as related vitamins, enzymes, and minerals—which act with the vitamin to ensure that it is absorbed and properly used . . .

Most commercially produced supplements contain vitamins that are either crystalline or synthetic. Crystalline vitamins are those that have been separated from natural sources by chemical means; synthetic vitamins are produced "from scratch" in the laboratory. Both are purified or fractionated concentrates of the vitamin, which act more like drugs than nutrients in the body. They can actually disrupt the body chemistry and cause many imbalances.

Nourishing Traditions: The Cookbook that Challenges Politically Correct Nutrition and the Diet Dictocrats by S. Fallon and M. Enig, amzn.to/nB9irS

In fact, many vitamin and mineral supplements contain artificial additives, synthetic flow agents and chemical colorings that can easily cause reactions in your body.

Eat whole foods and cleanse your body, and you will absorb what you need from your food. Personally test any vitamins and minerals you want to take. Get sun. Add cod liver oil, which is a food, to your diet.

Use the following sources of information to find foods rich in the vitamins and minerals you want (caveat, a few of the foods are not in my "good" list, like soy): *Food Sources for Vitamins and Minerals* (tiny.cc/cnbzzw), *What Foods Have What Vitamins?* (tiny.cc/4nbzzw)

If you must have minerals, check out these high quality bioavailable ones: Kornax (bit.ly/nHUlMp)

Also, whenever you consider taking a vitamin or mineral supplement, make sure it is made from natural ingredients. Those "experts" who profess that natural or synthetic ingredients are all the same need to read this article: *Synthetic vs. Natural Vitamins* (tiny.cc/qfczzw).

The supplements may be chemically the same, but the effects on the body of the synthetic supplements can be quite different and in some cases very dangerous. The same risks occur in modern foods that add synthetic vitamins or minerals to raise the nutritional profiles. Be very wary of these non-foods. Over time they have a definite health destroying reaction.

Possible Supplements for You—Endogenous and Exogenous

Supplements that are found in common foods or naturally in our bodies are called "endogenous" supplements. Those that are **not** found in our bodies or in common foods are called "exogenous" supplements.

Basically, every food and their derivatives are endogenous, while many herbs are exogenous meaning they lose their benefits after 1–6 months, and you may have reactions to them (if not sooner!).

So when you come across a supplement or herb that you believe may be useful to you, personally test it and retest often. That is the only way to know if a suggestion is going to be good for you. If you get a YES response and the supplement is exogenous, know that you must stop using it at some point. I guarantee you that you will receive a NO test response at some point, and when you do just stop using it.

Some Possible Daily Supplements

Many manufacturers use a multitude of herbs for health supplements or as general antioxidants. The main ones can be seen in a table on the following page:

Supplement	Benefits
Beta Glucan	Antioxidant
Quercitin	Antioxidant
N-Acetyl-Cysteine	Antioxidant
CoQ10	Antioxidant
Lipoic Acid	Antioxidant
Food Enzymes and Probiotics	Digestive aid
FOS	Digestive aid
Acidophilus	Digestive aid
L-Glutamine	Digestive aid
Aloe Vera Juice	Digestive aid
Glucosamine	For bones and joints
PS (Phosphatidyl Serine)	Brain/memory supplement
Acetyl-L-Carnitine	Health enhancer
Flax Oil	Omega-3 fatty acids (cod liver oil is a good alternative)
Lecithin	Protects against many diseases

Specific Prostate Supplements

There are many interesting herbal prostate products on the market today. Most prostate supplements come in capsule form and some as tinctures or teas. You will find many of the ingredients listed below as well as many added vitamins and minerals and some superfood greens.

The common practice is "the more, the better." I am not so sure about that, as it is easy to have a negative reaction to one or more of the ingredients, especially given what we now know about the dangers of vitamin supplementation by non-food sources. I find taking simpler versions gives me a YES test response sometimes when I test, while the concoctions give me a NO. You will have to test to decide.

Prostate Supplement	Benefits
Beta-Sitosterol/ Phytosterols	The active ingredient in Saw Palmetto.
Saw Palmetto	The best known prostate herb; many studies show that it's a preventative and helps to reduce prostate symptoms.
Pygeum	Another well-known prostate herb; many studies show its benefits for an enlarged prostate.
Nettle leaves	Very popular in Europe to treat BPH; often combined with saw palmetto to relieve BPH symptoms: urgency to urinate, incomplete emptying and constant urge to urinate.
Pumpkin seed extract	Contains high levels of phytates, so be careful
Lycopene	Conflicting research on this one . . . some say it is a useless ingredient
Soy Isoflavones	Mixed reviews on this one as with soy in general with some saying it is essential for prostate health
Zinc	A crucial prostate mineral: best to eat oysters and other zinc foods (brazil nuts, wild salmon, liver, egg yolks, sea salt, dark maple syrup)
DIM (a phytochemical produced while digesting cruciferous vegetables)	Lowers excess estrogens (eat cruciferous veggies)
Pollens	Like rye pollen and others
Small Willow Herb (epilobium parviflorum)	Common in Europe
Selenium	An important mineral deficient in our soils

If you are relatively healthy and have only minor symptoms, you may not have any negative reactions to a broad-spectrum prostate supplement. It may work well for you. If you have a more serious condition, then a simpler version or single herb may be the way to go.

Mother Nature Prostate Formulas

Prostate supplements at Amazon

Saw Palmetto is the most common prostate herb. Some men get relief from using it. Trust your personal test results no matter how incredible the fancy marketing brochures appear! Some claim the whole herb is the best way to go, while others suggest you take the active ingredient in it, as that is more potent.

There can be a world of difference between a whole herb, such as Saw Palmetto, and an isolated and concentrated nutrient taken from it, such as Beta Sitosterol, which often gets promoted as way more potent than the herb itself. I seriously question that assertion because it could be the interaction of different nutrients in the whole herb that is most powerful. Look at this recent article:

> *The synergy in which phytochemicals affect the human body is complex. Synthetically produced phytochemicals, or nutrients used as pharmaceuticals, do not have the same action as those naturally occurring in the whole food. Plant foods contain a synergy of nutrients and phytochemicals that have potent anti-cancer actions, along with antioxidant and other health promoting effects on the body. The importance of these foods in the diet is undisputed; however, the reductionist medical view of turning nature's perfect food into pharmaceutical drugs misses the point. When isolating compounds unforeseen actions can occur and side effects begin to emerge where they are not seen when consuming the whole plant.*

> *Researchers Believe Plant Based Food Could be Used as an Effective Treatment for Cancer by T. M. Hartle,* tiny.cc/snczzw

Dr. Andrew Weil wrote an insightful article on the differences between whole plants and the drugs that are isolated from them:

> *Using whole-plant remedies is a fundamentally different—and, I would argue, often better—way to treat illness . . . Human beings and plants have co-evolved for millions of years, so it makes perfect sense that our complex bodies would be adapted to absorb needed, beneficial compounds from complex plants and ignore the rest. This is an established fact in nutrition, but the West's sharp distinction between food and medicine somehow blinds us to these properties when it comes to botanicals . . . Plants are (usually) better than pharmaceutical drugs.*

> *Why Plants Are (Usually) Better than Drugs by Dr. A. Weil,* tiny.cc/umczzw

For a good tincture of just 3 ingredients, try *Prostate Doctor–Native Remedies* (bit.ly/qyIRWj). I like tinctures for their direct absorption. I also really like this very high quality tincture, Men's Formula, by Baseline Nutritionals (tiny.cc/kqczzw).

Another good quality Ayurvedic prostate supplement is *Prostate Protection—A Holistic Approach to Prostate Health* (tiny.cc/jsczzw).

The only way you will know for sure is by personally testing each supplement. (I know I say this a lot, but if you want to save time and lots of money, then personal testing cannot be beat!)

Here is a fascinating supplement, *Prostex*, I just discovered doing some research (amzn.to/nfd6Pe).

> *Amino acids are the building blocks of protein, and occur naturally in the body. Prostatic fluid has been found to contain particularly high concentrations of the amino acids glycine, alanine, and glutamic acid, and a special formula of these three substances has been used for decades to treat the urinary symptoms of BPH . . .*
>
> *While the exact method of action is not fully understood, it is thought that, like other nutritional and herbal supplements, the formula works through a diuretic and anti-edemic effect, reducing excess swelling of prostate and surrounding tissues and encouraging normal urine flow."*
>
> *Amino Acid Therapy by Prostex*, tiny.cc/duczzw

Order on their site or here at Amazon, which is a bit cheaper: *Advanced Prostex* (tiny.cc/u2c3a).

Here is a great high density potent supplement you can try: *Prost-P10x*. This one stands out. Why? Because of the quality and amount of ingredients. They come in an individual day pack inside the bottle. You will find cheaper but none better (tiny.cc/cwczzw).

Check out this high potency phytosterol/beta-sitosterol product: NeoProstate (tiny.cc/3yczzw).

My bottom line on prostate supps: they may be helpful for a period but my experience is that they provide diminishing returns while the highest quality foods seem to supply augmenting returns. Be careful and test!

Here is a source for French Green Clay Capsules (bit.ly/oMsrBu) that Is an inexpensive supplement that also acts as a cleanser to remove toxins from the body:

> *While many people recognize the benefits of natural clays for skincare, most Americans have yet to experience the age-old European practice of including specialized French Green Clay in the diet. This special form of clay (also known as illite clay) features minerals, trace elements and phytonutrients (which give it its green color). It also absorbs unwanted substances in the GI tract, making it an excellent addition to any detoxification program.*
>
> *Swanson Premium French Green Clay Natural Detoxifier by Swanson Health Products* (tiny.cc/y1czzw)

Use the following anti-inflammatory herbs in your cooking if they test YES: rosemary, cinnamon, oregano, turmeric, ginger and garlic.

Eat zinc-rich foods like oysters and properly prepared nuts and seeds. Many men are very deficient in zinc, as much as 30-50% of men; the deficiency is worse the older you are. This is a prime driver of prostate problems.

Eat wild not farmed salmon regularly for its omega-3 fatty acids.

Eat cruciferous vegetables (a natural source of DIM used in some supplements) like broccoli, cabbage, Brussels sprouts, kale, bok choy, su choy, collard greens and broccoli sprouts.

> *Sulforaphane from broccoli and cruciferous vegetables selectively destroys cancer cells.*
>
> *Research details published in the Molecular Nutrition & Food Research journal explains the potent mechanism exhibited by . . . broccoli and cauliflower to ameliorate developing cancer cells. The active photochemical known as sulforaphane targets prostate and other hormone dependent cancer lines and leaves normal healthy cells unaffected.*
>
> *Sulforaphane from Broccoli and Cruciferous Vegetables Selectively Destroys Cancer Cells by J. Phillip,* tiny.cc/l3czzw

Other Herbs for the Prostate

Herbs can detox and cleanse the prostate gland, and they can reduce swelling and inflammation by dissolving toxins within the gland. Try some of these:

Peppermint

Peppermint—not spearmint—acts as an anti-inflammatory to the prostate. It may be a useful tea.

Turmeric

This curry spice and herb is an anti-inflammatory. It is available in capsules.

Here are some other prostate herbs:

- Cleavers herb
- Thuja leaf
- Juniper berries
- Corn silk
- Willow herbs (Epilobium parviflorum)- very commonly prescribed in Europe
- Great hairy willow herb (E. hirsutum)
- Uva ursi leaves
- Horsetail (Equisetum arvense)
- Sweet and spotted Joe-Pye rhizome (Eupatorium purpureum and E. maculatum)
- Rye pollen
- Queen Ann's lace (Daucus carota)
- Yellow and white sweet clover herb (Melilotus officinalis and M. alba)

Herbal Prostate Tea

Bell Prostate Ezee Flow Tea is an herbal prostate tea that many men swear by (tiny.cc/v4czzw).

Chinese Herbs and Products

You will find many Chinese herbs for the prostate if you search for them. I would look for a product that contains some of the herbs listed on the website below but with my usual caveats—personally test everything (see Chapter 9).

Prostate Health—How to Treat and Prevent Enlarged Prostate with Chinese Herbs (tiny.cc/i6czzw)

Here are some other Chinese herbal products:

Chinese Prostate Supplement (bit.ly/nFvNXP)

Chinese Herbs for Prostate (tiny.cc/ekmzzw)

There is a long tradition of herbal healing in China passed down over the generations. If you live near a Chinatown, then I recommend that you see a Chinese herbal doctor. Just go into various herbal stores and ask them for a Chinese herbal doctor. They will direct you. I have done this on several occasions.

The Chinese herbal doctor will take your pulses to learn your condition and examine your tongue and more as well as ask you questions about your health and diet. From that examination, the Chinese herbal doctor will customize an herbal product for you. It will be weighed and mixed with a variety of herbs with instructions on how to simmer them to make a tonic to drink over the next week or two. Depending on your condition, this can be a very effective treatment for your prostate.

If you do not live near a Chinatown, then you could get an email consultation at *Dr. Shen's Chinese Herbs and Medicine.* Scroll to the bottom of this page: tiny.cc/ekmzzw.

Herbs work differently from strong medications, which often have dangerous side effects. Herbs work slowly, cleansing and rebuilding, and are more subtle in their effects, but they do have a powerful impact over time. Just because they are herbs does not mean they are good for you! Many will not be so the only thing to do is TEST.

Conclusion

My advice is rather than supplement, purchase the best quality foods that you can. If you do choose to supplement your diet, use bioavailable natural supplements made from whole foods and herbs, definitely avoid synthetic versions and personally test before consuming. Even better, save yourself a lot of money and test before making the purchase!

In Chapter 9, I finally share my knowledge and experience about personal testing.

Chapter 9: Personal Testing

Wouldn't it be wonderful to have a reliable way to **know** whether something is healthy for you to eat or use? And to just **know** that you know! In fact, there are simple techniques you can learn that can give you those answers.

Caveat: the techniques to which I'm referring will be very challenging for many readers to accept, especially those of you with a very scientific mindset. I know that personal testing could be easily dismissed as unscientific and not valid.

That would be a mistake.

Why? Because I know it works.

I have had countless examples of being able to discover a problematic food or supplement, which within hours of taking it, caused me very severe reactions including complete inability to urinate. It would have been far better to have tested that item before ingesting it and thus avoiding the problem.

I am a slow learner sometimes, and I have paid the price for that weakness. But I have always been able to find the culprit afterwards by testing all that I ate in my last meal. And many times I have stopped myself from taking something that personally tested NO and thus was able to avoid those reactions.

Suspend your judgment if you want results! Personal testing works if done correctly. If you have a prostate condition, then testing your inputs is a crucial step to stop the triggers that are worsening your condition.

I call it "personal testing" because you are testing whether something is beneficial for you or not. It has other names as well: muscle testing, behavioral kinesiology, body tuning, energy testing, energy awareness, bio-energetic testing, bio-resonance, pendulum testing, personal dowsing and more. If you have heard these terms before and have negative thoughts about them, please suspend your judgment and read on.

Personal testing can quickly let you know:

- whether a food is good for you or not,
- whether a supplement is conducive to your health or not,
- whether a medication or herbal remedy is good for you or not,
- whether a body care product is good for you or not,
- whether a household product is conducive to your health, or not, and
- how much of an item is optimum to take.

Here's an example: I love chocolate! I have not been able to test positive for months and months. I go into the health food store and test their organic chocolates, and I always get a NO, no matter how much I wish for a YES! I gave up testing chocolate for about a month and, lo and behold, I am now getting a YES for a small amount of 85% dark organic chocolate.

There are no theories or facts about what you should or shouldn't eat. All you need to do is be patient with yourself as you attempt to learn to personally test foods and products.

It takes a bit of time, but with persistence, you will develop a skill that is invaluable to have for your health.

What is Personal Testing?

Personal testing involves tapping into your personal awareness or bio-energy by learning to center into your subconscious, which then gives you the answer you are seeking.

We all have that internal guidance system. It comes with being human. In an article entitled *The Intelligence of Your Cells*, Dr. Bruce Lipton stated that the conscious mind is capable of processing 40 nerve impulses per second (tiny.cc/jpmzzw). The subconscious mind can process 40,000,000 nerve impulses per second! Hence, when you personally test, you tap into your inner knowing—subconscious mind—and bring it to conscious awareness.

We all have the ability. The problem is that many of us have lost the ability to tap directly into our inner knowing. Modern life disconnects us from our roots with nature and puts stresses of all kinds on us. The list of reasons that we are disconnected goes on and on.

How many times in your life have you said to yourself, "I'm full, I shouldn't eat any more," and then found yourself dishing up yet another plateful of food? You didn't listen to your body and ate more anyway. The discomfort from being overfull and overfed is ignored.

In the West, we have trained ourselves to stop listening to our bodies' signals and needs. We ignore the feedback mechanisms that are meant to keep us healthy and in balance.

Personal testing gives you a way to tap into that inner wisdom and to learn to listen to what is right for you in this moment. This will help you choose foods and products that are truly health enhancing to help prevent health problems, to speed you on the path to recovery and to heal your prostate if you have a condition.

Some readers may scoff at the techniques for personal testing, possibly because they think it is not scientific. What I can tell you is this: It has worked for me and for thousands of others—there is no cost or drawback to giving this a try.

With an open mind, try the techniques outlined in this chapter. Try it in the quiet comfort of your home, with no one watching, and see what happens. If these techniques work for you, then you have gained an unparalleled tool that will facilitate your health and save you time and money. There is nothing to lose and everything to gain.

All I can say to you, dear reader, is that this skill has saved me from countless agonizing experiences and has speeded me to recovery from a very unhappy prostate. If you are able to put aside your doubts and skepticism and give this an honest try, I believe it will be a boon for you. It will take time and effort to get good at it, but it is worth doing, believe me!

Luckily there are three basic ways to do personal testing, one of which will work well for you.

How to Personally Test

Three basic personal testing techniques that you can use are:

1. muscle testing with a partner,
2. personal muscle testing and
3. pendulum testing.

Eventually, as your awareness develops and your natural instincts and intuition are strengthened, you may simply know whether something is beneficial for you or not without using testing techniques.

Personally, since I am a very visual person, I love seeing the results of a test and find pendulum testing my favorite. Others who may be more attuned to sensations may find personal muscle testing to be their favorite, while others may enjoy and find they get the best response when testing with a partner.

Whichever test you end up attuning to, let yourself practice more and more. Tell your inner skeptic to take a sabbatical while you test drive personal testing—the benefits are so worthwhile! You can save yourself a lot of pain and even help prevent prostate attacks!

Personal testing will also save you a lot of money because you won't buy products that may be wonderful for others, but not for you (at least at this time). You will be able to design your own perfect diet, not one based on some expert's advice (including me!).

I offer you these three methods so that you can find one that you like. There are slight variations on each. Just develop the skill with whichever works best for you. Okay, let's begin!

Muscle Testing with a Partner:

Also known as behavioral kinesiology, this test requires two people: you and your partner, who will test you. The environment should be quiet and calm.

1. Both of you stand. Your left arm should hang down comfortably at your side. Your dominant arm (for most people it is their right arm) extends outward in a horizontal position with your elbow fully extended. (If you are left-handed, reverse the arms.)

2. Your partner should stand behind you. Close your eyes and relax your mind. Your partner then places her left hand on your left shoulder to keep you stable, and the fingers of her right hand on top of your right arm over your wrist. Some prefer to face each other, but I think it is best to avoid visual contact.

3. Your partner will say, "Resist," and then press down quickly on your arm while you try to resist the pressure. Your partner should do this firmly and smoothly. It is not a contest but rather a way to notice if the arm remains strong or weakens.

4. Your arm muscle will test strong in this neutral state. If you are in an emotional state or under the influence of drugs or alcohol, it is not a good time to test as you could get mixed results.

5. Now we want to test something true. Your partner will ask, "Is your name [insert your name]?" Your arm should remain strong, which is a YES response.

6. Now your partner will ask a question that will give a negative response, such as, "Is your name Mary?" Your arm will become weak and will descend when pushed down on, which is a NO response.

Now you are ready to test a food or product. Hold the food item in your non-dominant hand (for most people this is the left hand) against your prostate area or solar plexus. Then repeat the arm test. If the product is good for you, your arm will remain strong; if your arm is weak and it collapses, then the product is not good for you at this time. Now you have your answer!

In the case of a supplement that gave you a YES response, you then want to know how much to take. Here is what to do. Start with one capsule in the palm of your hand and test again. If you get a YES, then try 2, then 3. Keep testing until you get a NO. The last YES is your dose for the day. You could take that amount spread over the day (e.g., take one supplement three times if you have three capsules as the daily dose).

In the case of a food like eggs that tested YES, retest with one egg then 2, and so on, to see how many you can eat.

It is wise to retest an item every day to ensure that it is still valid or that the dose doesn't change; this is especially important when you begin using new products. For example, I started testing a new supplement that gave me a YES response. The label advised 2 capsules per day, but I tested for 8! I obviously needed that supplement (cod liver oil)! That dosage lasted for a week. Through repeated testing, I started to reduce the dose per day down to 2 and then 1 capsule. And then for a while, none.

You will have to practice the testing until it becomes easy and natural to you. It is necessary to have an open and calm mind when you do muscle testing. Remember your inner critic is AWL (away with leave)!

This *Muscle Testing with a Partner* video is good to watch because it demos the basic technique (tiny.cc/ctn2zw).

Your arm muscles will respond to a particular item either with weakness or with strength, so long as you test properly. Many foods and health products that seem irresistible based on their nutritious contents and marketing will test NO. I find that some wonderful products do this. If you test NO for a product that seems to have many "good" ingredients, it may be because one of the ingredients does not resonate for you. Trust your test results. Move on to something else. Your body may not be able to process or digest it properly, and you do not want to weaken your condition.

Personal Muscle Testing

If you don't have a partner to help you, you can still muscle test alone. There are two ways to do this:

Standing Method

Stand in a relaxed manner and repeat the word "YES" to yourself. Allow your body to move or swing you forward. Now repeat the word "NO," and you will find your whole body moving backwards. Thus, by holding a food or supplement against your prostate area, you will either tilt forward or backward, depending on your body's response to it. Does it resonate or not?

Try the name test: My name is [use your name]. You should swing forward a bit—YES. Then say something false: "My name is [use someone else's name]." The opposite now—NO. You don't need to make the statements aloud—silently is fine. The idea is to train your mind for truth and falsehood, YES and NO. Just practice this for a few minutes a day until it works for you.

Try some seemingly obvious items: see if Coke gives you a YES or NO and then try an orange or carrot. You are ready to test now!

Here is a link to a video for the *Standing Personal Muscle Test* (tiny.cc/8un2zw).

Finger Method

Hold the thumb and first finger of your left hand so they make a circle (reverse if you are left handed). With the index finger of your right hand, you place it inside the circle and say YES, then pull it briskly outward (towards where your thumb and index finger are connected). You should test strong (YES), and you will not be able to open the circle. Now do it with NO and your finger should open the circle.

Do the same name test as above to get your YES and NO responses. Now you are ready to test.

You can then hold the product you want to test against your prostate area or sternum using your arm while you then use your fingers to test. If it is a negative product, your finger will open and exit the circle.

Some testers use different fingers. Use what seems best for you. Here is a video for the *Finger Personal Muscle Test* (tiny.cc/wwmzzw).

Pendulum Testing

Pendulum testing is my favorite, and I also believe it can be the most accurate method if used correctly. Pendulum testing requires the use of a pendulum to see your YES and NO responses. What I particularly like is that there is a way to ensure you do not get a false test, like a false positive. That technique will ensure optimum accuracy of your results.

Pendulum testing amplifies your body's awareness and responses to what you are testing.

While a pendulum can be made out of virtually any object that you can hang off of a string, there are better and more responsive pendulums that you can purchase. I believe that getting the best pendulum is well worth the price of around $30—the best purchase of my life!

You will instantly break-even the first time you go to buy a supplement that is supposedly great for you, and you test and get a NO. You will then have recovered the price of the pendulum, and it's free sailing from then on.

To avoid false positives and personal reactions to the device itself, select a pendulum that mimics the shape of the body's energy field, which is egg-like. This eliminates many pendulums offered for sale in shops and Internet sites.

The most responsive and accurate device is called the Perfect Pendulum. The people who make and sell Perfect Pendulums are experts in the field of personal energy testing with decades of experience, and I highly recommend these as they are the very best.

Once you master using the pendulum you can then graduate to using your body or hands as the testing device, even more accurately than the above methods. I still have a personal liking for seeing the responses, so I use my pendulum every time I test.

I can easily test with an old nail, nail clippers or exotic drop-shape pendulums with points on the bottom. I have used them all, but none come close to the accuracy and ease of a Perfect Pendulum.

The detailed instructions that come with the Perfect Pendulum are equally as valuable as the pendulum itself. These instructions describe how to use the Perfect Pendulum for different kinds of testing that I have never seen done accurately with the other testing methods. Keep in mind that you cannot ask just any question when testing with a pendulum. This technique requires getting a direct YES or NO response.

Being made of opaque stone, the Perfect Pendulums are more accurate than glass, wood, plastic or other materials, which helps to avoid switching errors (i.e., when your energy switches back and forth, which will affect your testing responses).

The following information is from the Perfect Pendulum website (bit.ly/m7J913):

1. *Hold the chain between your thumb and index finger, with the small ball in your palm.*

2. *Deliberately swing the pendulum backwards and forwards with your wrist dropped rather than straight.*

3. *Have the flat palm of your free hand facing up.*

4. *While watching your pendulum, touch your thumb and index finger together—this is called acceptance mudra.*

   If your pendulum veers into a circle, this is your YES direction

   If it doesn't, open your fingers, wait a few seconds, start the pendulum swinging back and forth again, then close thumb and index finger again while watching your pendulum. Each time you do this, you are clearing your bio-energetic testing circuit

   Continue doing this until you get a change of direction with acceptance mudra.

Once you have found your YES direction, you should also practice your NO direction. This is exactly the same process, using acceptance mudra again, but with your palm facing down this time.

Please note: it's very important that you generate your YES and NO directions with the acceptance mudra. Other techniques, such as writing YES and NO on different pieces of paper or asking yourself questions, should not be used.

Testing for switching—the self test: *Before doing any sort of energy testing (with your pendulum, a muscle test etc.), you must first establish whether your energetic 'testing circuits' are flowing properly. Your energies can 'switch' often during the day, perhaps as a reaction to a food, a person or being in a certain place. So it is very important to check yourself before using your body as a testing instrument—which is what you are doing when using a pendulum. Many people use pendulums without checking to see if their body is working properly and hence get false or variable results. You can only evaluate the correctness of your answer using a pendulum, if you know that you are reliably getting a 'YES' or a 'NO'.*

To do the Self Test, place the Self Test mudra—the thumb pointing out between the two middle fingers of your closed fist—against your heart center. The heart center is approximately two inches up from the bottom of your sternum (breast bone).

A NO means 'not switched', no problems, you can test. A YES means you are switched and must unswitch your circuits before you can use the pendulum or do a muscle test.

Perfect Pendulums Information by The School of Energy Awareness (bit.ly/m7J913)

If you test "switched," just follow the instructions to unswitch. Now that you can get a YES or NO, this is the way I test a product or food. I hold the item against my prostate area and test by swinging the pendulum forwards and back and then it will give me a YES or NO by the direction it then rotates. It's as simple as that.

Below I share with you two videos I made demonstrating personal testing. Before you see these videos, I want to caution you that the motions of your pendulum may be very subtle at the beginning. The turning won't be as strong for you as you see in these videos demonstrating how I personally test foods and products. It may take time for your responses to become as powerful as mine, but even a small movement YES or NO is enough to get your answer.

Part 1: *Pendulum Personal Testing* (tiny.cc/20mzzw)

Part 2: *Pendulum Personal Testing* (tiny.cc/x1mzzw)

Occasionally, you will get a neutral response, neither a yes nor a no. Nothing happens or what happens is unclear. That means exactly that: the product is neither good nor bad. If you are healthy, then use that product in moderation. If you have a health condition, then I would not use that product unless you feel there is a good reason. When you are stronger, then it will not matter as much. Retest that item later if you want to use it again.

If you find you are having difficulties learning to personally test products then go to Food Energy Awareness Solutions and Training for an online consultation with the experts. These experts can help you learn with specific tips or by testing the foods and supplements that you want. Stephen and Lynda Kane are exceptional in this area. They are the ones who taught me and are the makers of the pendulum that I use.

Another solution is to get the book *Diet Wise* by Dr. Scott-Mumby (tiny.cc/x1mzzw). You won't need to know how to test but by eliminating many foods, and then adding them back one at a time, you can see which ones trigger a reaction. This will be much harder and more lengthy to do but will work.

Here is another option for you. Take this survey of symptoms (tiny.cc/e5mzzw). The company will then test 115 foods to find your culprits. But this is far inferior to learning how to personally test.

Personal testing will revolutionize and empower your life.

Try to Set Aside Your Skepticism

I know, it's a bit too wacky for you and over the edge! This writer is too much!

But our subconscious knows what is best for us. Testing just tunes you into a conscious awareness of what you already know.

I know it is surprising, but this approach has consistently worked for me. Many times I've tested an unopened product in a health food store and then retested the same product at home with the actual capsule in my hand, and I got the same response.

Personal testing has also worked on something that I sure wished was a YES, but I got a NO response. It was a super sounding prostate supplement, and I wanted to try it, but NO means NO so I passed on it.

On many occasions, I have bought something from the Internet that tested YES from the product image and that still tested the same when it arrived. The last time I did it, I tested the package without opening it after I got it all wrapped from the post office. Then I tested it in the bottle. All times were a YES, including the pill itself.

At times, I have taken a supplement that I didn't or forgot to test because it sounded so good! But later it caused a reaction. My typical reactions are either a sore tongue or frequent urination or worse – none, usually within hours, which indicates a prostate reaction. Then later, I test the supplement and get a NO. If only I had tested sooner!

If you have concerns about a bias or having an agenda, then consider muscle testing with a partner (as shown earlier in this chapter). If you have concerns about people seeing you attempt this in a store, try the Finger Method (also shown earlier in this chapter), as this approach can be very subtle. It looks like you're fidgeting, and no one will even notice you doing it. Frankly, I don't care. I use my pendulum wherever! Most people do not even notice you—they are too concerned with their own shopping.

I know it is hard to put your skepticism aside, but you have nothing to lose and a lot to gain. Try it and see! This has worked like a charm for me and saved me countless dollars, and I hope it works for you too.

Your body's inner wisdom knows what it needs and what you need constantly changes as seasons change, as you change, as your body heals and grows, as certain foods no longer serve you and new foods are needed.

Let's take an example: coffee. Many pundits say it is terrible for you, and others claim that its antioxidants will cure what ails you! So how are you to know? By personally testing, you will get a clear answer for you right now. At the time of this writing, I test YES for organic coffee and NO for the often touted, the-more-you-drink-the-better green tea! In fact, if I drink green tea my body starts reacting to it, and my frequency of urination goes way up while the opposite happens with caffeinated coffee. Go figure!

So who are you to believe? Some guru pundit or your body's own inner wisdom? I know my answer and so will you when you learn how to tune in to your inner subconscious body wisdom.

How do I know personal testing works?

Because I "back-tested" it. I believe my extreme sensitivities to many foods developed because my gut flora had weakened from

- vaccines, which weaken your body;
- antibiotics, which destroy good flora;
- mercury fillings, which leak minute amounts of highly toxic mercury into the body; and
- the anti-nutrient, phytic acid, in many whole natural foods.

I used to wake up in the middle of the night unable to pee—totally blocked! I eventually learned something had triggered the shutdown.

The way that I back-tested was by personal testing everything I had eaten at supper time. I always found something that tested NO—the culprit! And so I started to test foods before I ate them. (That was a simple brain wave!)

I had to give up all that I had learned about diet and the supposedly healthy foods with great profiles and scientific research. The only thing that mattered to me was whether I would react to it—or not.

Real foods like my own garden kale, freshly picked, or apples from my own trees—and many more simple foods—could block me tight so I had to use a catheter to pee! These natural wholesome foods were also culprits at some point: zucchini, beets, organic dairy unless raw, rice and bread, coffee, green tea, all herbal teas and almost all supplements!

Because my symptoms were so observable and so immediate, I became a living laboratory. My health was revolutionized by being able to personally test foods and supplements even of the highest quality and by discovering that many of them would not work for me.

By stopping all the irritants, I was finally able to stop the downslide and begin to heal. Now I can eat many of those former trigger foods—no problem!

Without personal testing, my condition probably would have worsened.

Personal testing is the most important health discovery of all time in my opinion because it allows you to know what works for you—no theories, no guesswork, no must do's. You know. Period.

Personal Testing Theory

If you want to learn how this works, read more here: *Energy Medicine* (tiny.cc/76mzzw) or *Muscle Testing* (tiny.cc/2g1fb). And this book, *Blinded by Science*, explains many mysteries of nature so you can understand how it works as well (www.blindedbyscience.co.uk/).

How personal testing works through a closed package or bottle is a mystery to me, but again it does work. I can live with uncertainty about how it works because it has proven, without a shadow of a doubt, to work for me. It removes all the guesswork from my choices about other experts' recommendations. I just personally test each item and get my answer.

Testing Tips

When you get a YES for something new, retest it again regularly to ensure that the product is still good for you, especially if you have many sensitivities or if you are healing. You can calm your mind by placing your tongue up to touch the roof of your mouth behind your top teeth (an advanced meditation technique). Then test. When you get good at testing, it will only take a few seconds to get a response.

Remember no matter how "good" for you a food or supplement is, whether recommended in this book or elsewhere, if you have too much of it, then it can easily change to "bad" for you! It has happened to me many times—with ghee, miso, sauerkraut, saw palmetto, selenium, greens, flax oil and more!

As you cleanse, detox and start to heal, your sensitivity to foods and supplements goes up. Your body knows what it needs. Set aside your opinions and personally test (and retest). You will then know what is healthy for you to eat or not. As you get healthier and your sensitivity diminishes, you find that you have fewer reactions.

Conclusion

Each one of us is so unique that we need these tools to **know** what is best for us. It is easy to learn one (or more) of these tests, and this skill will empower you to make the right health decisions for you.

Personal testing will revolutionize your health by going beyond the advice and recommendations of others—no matter how qualified or eminent they are. Testing goes beyond the selling points of a product or the ideas someone else has for you about what you "need" or what you "should" eat. Testing allows you to know for sure.

Take all the good advice that comes your way and put it to good use by testing and making decisions based on your true knowing.

Chapter 10: Conclusion

We live in a world of great complexity and have the benefit in the West of access to a wide range of foods and supplements. The keys to health are to embrace a diet rich in whole natural foods and nutrients, to learn how to prepare foods using time tested traditional methods that enhance digestibility and vitamin mineral absorption, and to supplement wisely with the highest quality natural ingredients that you personally test to reveal a need in your body.

By doing these things, you will avoid the mistake that so many men make of thinking that more is better when they are actually harming themselves because they do not know what is best for them nor what their specific and unique dietary needs are.

Lastly, remember, you must stop those foods that trigger your condition and replace them with healthy ones that nourish you and your prostate. There are no shortcuts. Just good changes and little by little you will get better and prevent chronic prostate problems.

My hope is that you have learned or gleaned some useful insights. For me it is easy to give up bad habits, uninformed opinions and advice from pundits. When you know the impact on your health, it's easy to start discovering real foods and to give up unhealthy manufactured concoctions.

When you find your prostate health diet, you are ensured not only great prostate health but overall vitality for years of benefits.

> *"If you enjoyed reading this book, I'd appreciate it if you would take a couple of minutes to post a short review at Amazon. Intelligent reviews help other customers make better buying choices. And because I read all my reviews personally, they will help me to write better books in the future. Thanks for your support!"*

Ron Bazar

Other Books and Websites by Ronald M. Bazar

Healthy Prostate: The Extensive Guide to Prevent and Heal Prostate Problems Including Prostate Cancer, BPH Enlarged Prostate and Prostatitis (tiny.cc/qanzzw)

Do You Know the 10 Worst Foods for Your Prostate Health? (tiny.cc/sbnzzw)

Prostate Health: Learn the 10 Amazing Functions of Your Prostate (tiny.cc/mcnzzw)

BeaBea: Her Diary Her Life: Beatrice Millman Bazar: Her diary from the summer of 1931 and highlights from the rest of her life (with Kaima Bazar) (tiny.cc/bdnzzw)

Good Planets are Hard to Find (with Roma Dehr) (tiny.cc/9dnzzw)

From A to Z by Bike (with Roma Dehr) (tiny.cc/4enzzw)

I Love Not Smoking: An Activity Book for Non Smoking Children (with Roma Dehr) (tiny.cc/tfnzzw)

Websites

www.ProstateHealthDiet.org

www.HealthyProstate.co

www.NaturalProstate.com

www.ArbutusArts.com

Made in the USA
Middletown, DE
15 December 2016